HEALTH LITERACY IN CONTEXT

INTERNATIONAL PERSPECTIVES

PUBLIC HEALTH IN THE 21ST CENTURY

Additional books in this series can be found on Nova's website
under the Series tab.

Additional e-books in this series can be found on Nova's website
under the E-book tab.

EDUCATION IN A COMPETITIVE
AND GLOBALIZING WORLD

Additional books in this series can be found on Nova's website
under the Series tab.

Additional e-books in this series can be found on Nova's website
under the E-book tab.

CONTENTS

PREFACE

Health literacy offers a new way of thinking about how we engage with information about and for health, both as users and providers of information. As a multifaceted construct, health literacy weaves together ideas drawn from health and adult education/literacy disciplines. The complexity of health literacy necessarily reflects the contexts in which it applies and the perspectives of those who integrate and examine it in their research and practice. This book captures the richness in thinking about health literacy by presenting perspectives of international researchers and practitioners who have been working on health literacy in diverse settings and contexts.

Chapter 1 - Health literacy is an important concept—one that this book considers in context and from different international perspectives. In this chapter, we introduce readers to the evolving concept of health literacy and present a timeline of key events from the first recorded mention of health literacy to the present. In addition, we look at health literacy as both an individual and systemic concern, with some scholars considering it from a clinical point of view and others from a public health or community empowerment view. The health literacy experts from the United States, the United Kingdom, Canada, China, Ireland, and Israel who presented at *Health Literacy: Making the Most of Health* conference that took place in London, England, in February 2010 later wrote the chapters that appear in this book. These chapters are on timely topics relevant to health literacy including definitions, healthy lifestyle, health outcomes, lifelong learning, culture and community, and economics.

Chapter 2 - In recent years, health literacy has emerged as a substantive and rich field of inquiry. However, there has not always been full agreement on what exactly is meant by the term *health literacy* itself. With health literacy increasingly considered a social determinant of health, focused attention to its definition is warranted. A definition not only sets parameters but also indirectly shapes questions for inquiry; it offers guidelines for measurement and, in the case of health literacy, indicates a locus of control and responsibility that may influence research, practice, and policy decisions. Early definitions of health literacy focused on the skills and abilities of individuals to gain access to, understand, and use information. However, attention has been increasingly focused on the assumptions and skills of those professionals who develop and provide health messages, directions, and information and on those institutions providing services and care. This growing attention to the physical and social contexts of health activities calls for renewed attention to the definition of health literacy with its focus on individuals. We argue that a more comprehensive definition of health literacy must include both the abilities of individuals and the characteristics of professionals and institutions that support or that may inhibit individual or community action. Any such definition will unquestionably need to be accompanied by measurement tools that fully operationalize its key concepts—thereby including not only measurements of the abilities of the lay public but also of the texts, of the skills of health professionals, and of the expectations and assumptions of health care environments.

Chapter 3 - Information intended to persuade people to make healthy lifestyle choices abounds from lay and professional, public and private sources within and beyond formal health systems. Positioning the relevant importance of the individual and the broader society in supporting personal health behaviours is central to public health policy and health literacy efforts aimed at improving health outcomes. This chapter examines the multidimensional concepts of health literacy and healthy lifestyle choices within two policy contexts, the United Kingdom and Canada, and from our respective fields of practice, pharmacy and nutrition. By drawing on the literature and examples from our research, we explore ideas about health literacy and the responsibility of individuals for using information to make and act upon an informed choice pertaining to their personal health behaviour.

Chapter 4 - In this chapter, we examine the impact of low health literacy on health outcomes. We review the body of research that has been published internationally, noting that the majority of these studies are describing simply the various associations between adult literacy skills and health outcomes rather than causation. Specifically, lack of reading fluency and low levels of health vocabulary (i.e., low literacy as applied to health) have been linked to problems with the use of preventive services, delayed diagnoses, understanding of one's medical condition, adherence to medical instructions, self-management skills, physical and mental health, and increased mortality risk. We consider what this evidence may say about possible causal pathways between health literacy and health outcomes and, very briefly, discuss the potential for interventions.

Chapter 5 - Health literacy is important throughout life and is, therefore, a crucial goal for lifelong learning both within and beyond formal educational settings. In turn, more educational involvement throughout life is correlated with an increase in health literacy, including the emerging concept of mental health literacy, and healthy behaviours. The basis for adult learning behaviours begins to be established in childhood and adolescence; however, learning through adulthood has a vitally important influence on health. Critical health literacy and empowerment arise from knowledge and skills in dealing proactively with health information. One promising example program, *Skilled for Health*, demonstrates various elements of health literacy and lifelong learning. Seniors who continue to engage in learning activities also improve their health. More research in lifelong learning and health literacy impact needs to include investigations of technology, especially as used by the commercial media and on the Internet; more research with adolescents; better measurement tools; knowledge translation (converting theoretical knowledge to practical application); and a more detailed understanding of mental health literacy.

Chapter 6 - This chapter explores the relationship between health literacy, culture and community. The notion of community with regard to health literacy focuses on groups within the population that identify themselves as having common culture, values, and/or needs and share a commitment to meeting them. The health literacy challenges of specific groups within communities (e.g., older adults, migrants, immigrants, and cultures in transition from traditional to western societies) are reviewed and discussed. The implications of virtual communities on health literacy are raised. Among these groups, navigating and making decisions related to the health system are emphasized. Examples of health literacy interventions among specific cultures in communities through literature review and case studies from the United Kingdom and Israel are presented. Gaps in present research are noted, particularly with regard to effectiveness of interventions; directions for future research and participatory action in the community are proposed.

Chapter 7 - A presentation at a 2009 Institute of Medicine health literacy workshop provides a conceptual framework to discuss the various economic angles of health literacy. To date, much of the research has focused on the skills and abilities of individuals with little attention paid to the other side of the *health literacy coin*—the demands/complexities of the health care system. This chapter examines both sides of the coin and uses the English health care system as a case study to illustrate an economic perspective of health literacy. The following questions are considered: Are health-literate individuals more efficient users of health care resources? Can we produce better health through investing in health literacy? Do health literacy interventions improve one's health outcomes? How does a third-party payer view health literacy? What incentive is there for a provider to advocate health literacy principles? How should a policy maker approach health literacy? The author concludes that it is imperative that the economic data requirements for decision making are understood and embraced by health literacy advocates.

Chapter 8 - In this concluding chapter, the Editors reflect on the unique opportunity presented by the sharing of interdisciplinary and international experiences and perspectives in the complex and important area of health literacy. We identify some key themes that flow through the chapters in the book, including the definitions and conceptions of health literacy and its measurement, issues of power, the impact of policy, and concern for health inequalities. Finally, we offer some conjectures about the future of health literacy and final questions for reflection for readers.

ACKNOWLEDGMENTS

The Editors wish to thank each of the chapter authors who contributed their time and expertise in creating this book. Their efforts and timely support reflected their personal commitment to advancing the emerging field of health literacy and their eagerness to share international perspectives. Special thanks to Irv Rootman for introducing the book to readers through his thoughtfully prepared Foreword.

The origins of this book lie in the presentations and conversations held at the *Health Literacy: Making the Most of Health* conference that took place in London, England, in February 2010. This conference was funded by the Department of Health (London) with additional sponsorship from the Food and Drink Federation (United Kingdom) and hosted by London South Bank University (London, United Kingdom), the University for Professional Opportunity. The conference was planned by members of the Health Literacy Group UK funded by the Department of Health (England) from 2007–2011.

The Editors are grateful to Shari Yore for her expertise and efficiency in copy and style editing this volume.

FOREWORD: CREATING BRIDGES WITH HEALTH LITERACY

Irving Rootman[*]

INTRODUCTION

Over the past decade of working with the concept of health literacy, I have become more and more impressed with the extent to which it facilitates the creation of bridges between different fields. Most obviously, it creates a bridge between health and education in that the concept itself embodies key outcomes in both fields. The concept also creates bridges within the health field itself and between those working in health care, health promotion, chronic disease prevention, rehabilitation medicine, and many other areas. This book, *Health Literacy in Context: International Perspectives*, makes it clear that work on health literacy is also capable of creating bridges between countries, as suggested by its subtitle, as well as by the process through which it was written with every chapter except one being co-authored by two or more people from different countries. Thus, as suggested in all of the chapters, although there are still many unmet challenges in the field of health literacy, we can meet them by working together across fields and countries and, in the process, continue to create bridges with one another.

My impression from reading the manuscript is that the 2010 *Health Literacy: Making the Most of Health* conference from which this emerged and

---

[*] irootman@telus.net.

the book itself have significantly advanced the creation of some of these bridges. Specifically, it appears to me that, as a result of the conference and this book, agreement and possibly consensus have emerged among a significant group of individuals in the field of health literacy on certain elements related to the concept as well as in directions for future progress.

POINTS OF AGREEMENT

Health Literacy is a Valuable Concept

First, it is clear that the authors of this book and likely most, if not all, participants in the conference agree that health literacy is in fact a valuable concept and deserves further attention and resources. This is not something that should be taken for granted; less than ten years ago, Keith Tones, a former editor of *Health Education Research*, argued that "there seems little if any justification for extending the original formulation of health literacy and incorporating it in re-packaged versions of existing theoretical formulations" (Tones, 2002, p. 289). I suspect that none of the authors of this book would agree with this statement—nor would the hundreds, if not thousands of researchers, practitioners, and policymakers and significant organizations that have undertaken work in relation to this concept since Tones made his comment.

Existing Definitions Have Limitations

Second, as is reflected in several chapters in this book, there appears to be agreement that none of the definitions of health literacy in current use are sufficiently comprehensive to encompass all important aspects of the concept. In particular, as Rudd, McCray, and Nutbeam argue in Chapter 2, existing and new definitions "do not fully address the capacity of health or health professionals to inhibit or enhance" the skills of individuals and communities emphasized in most definitions (p. 20). Whether or not there is an agreement—even among the authors that it is essential to have an international consensus on one comprehensive definition—is another matter. Indeed, Begoray, Rowlands, and Gillis suggest in the concluding chapter that the "freedom to choose and defend one's choice of definition is essential now and as the field of health literacy develops" (Chapter 8, p. 156), perhaps implying that we will never achieve international consensus. Nevertheless, I suspect that most, if not all, of the authors would agree with expanding the definition to include capacities of professionals and systems to support people and communities as well as with the need to give attention "to the logic and underlying assumptions inherent in the new and expanding definitions of health literacy" (Rudd et al., Chapter 2, p. 26).

Context is Critical

A third point of agreement is the importance of context in health literacy. This is not only emphasized in the chapter on definitions but also in the title of the book and in virtually all of the other chapters. Particular emphasis is given to it in the chapter on lifestyle choices as well as the chapter on culture and community. For example, Chapter 3 makes it clear that life choices or health behaviours that may result from health literacy cannot be understood without taking context into account. As Gillis and Gray state: "While it is recognized that personal behaviour can have a profound impact on one's health, these patterns and one's capacity for changing them depend heavily on circumstances of daily living" (Chapter 3, p. 34). In addition, they draw attention to the importance of the policy context by presenting case examples from two countries and note the relevance of ecological models that emphasize the importance of contexts. In Chapter 6, Levin-Zamir and Wells stress the critical importance of both culture and community in determining and supporting health literacy, especially in culturally and linguistically diverse communities, as well as the impact of health literacy in those contexts. They discuss the growing importance of virtual communities as a context for health literacy and present two case studies from the UK and Israel that illustrate the importance of context. Thus, although the authors of this book do not explicitly define the term *context*, Gillis, Begoray, and Rowlands do consider it to be "vital to the success of health literacy interventions" (Chapter 1, p. 2); and the book provides many examples of why this is so.

Existing Measures of Health Literacy Are Limited

The authors agree that the existing measures of health literacy are limited and that more appropriate measures need to be developed to measure contextual characteristics as well as the active engagement of people (Chapter

2). At the same time, it is acknowledged (Chapter 4) that some progress has been made in the development of measures and that using existing measures, limited as they are, we have learned a great deal about the positive impacts of greater health literacy and the negative impacts of less health literacy as well as about possible causal pathways between health literacy and health outcomes. Nevertheless, as Begoray et al. note, "more complex instruments are called for in both clinical and general health literacy decision-making contexts…" (Chapter 8, p. 157). They suggest that as the field evolves "we will need a variety of measures that both capture the wider range of skills inherent in more complex concepts and are sensitive to change." (Chapter 8, p. 158). Thus, it is clear that the issue of measurement needs to be given priority as we move forward. This, of course, is linked to the issue of definitions noted above and in Chapter 2.

A Life-course Perspective on Health Literacy is Important

A fifth area where there appears to be some agreement among the authors is the importance of taking a life-course perspective on health literacy. This is particularly prominent in Chapter 5, but it also appears in other chapters that mention age groups. In my view, this is certainly justified based not only on the arguments put forward by Begoray, Marshall, Shone, and Rowlands in Chapter 5 but also on the basis of a study in which I was involved that found that "education, lifelong and lifewide learning enabling factors exhibited the most robust associations with health literacy" (Wister, Malloy-Weir, Rootman, & Desjardins, 2010, p. 827). As suggested by Begoray et al., this is an area that clearly requires further research and one that has the potential for drawing in people working in the field of aging as well as education.

Health Literacy Contributes to and Addresses Inequities in Health

Although the authors do not use the term *inequities*, preferring to use the term *inequalities*, it is clear to me based on material in this book and other sources that health literacy both contributes to inequities (i.e., inequalities that are unfair) and is a means for reducing such inequities. For example, in Chapter 4 Protheroe, Wolf, and Lee note that research in the field has found that certain population groups such as those with lower socioeconomic status, ethnic minorities, older adults, and people with disabilities are more likely to have lower levels of health literacy than relevant comparison groups. They cite evidence that low health literacy is associated with a higher prevalence of certain chronic conditions (e.g., diabetes) as well as poorer physical and mental health, which are also higher in these groups. The extent to which health literacy "causes" the elevated negative health outcomes in disadvantaged groups is still to be determined, but it seems likely that it makes a contribution—thus, suggesting that it is a contributor to inequitable health inequalities.

This led this book's editors in the final chapter to conclude that: "Within clinical settings, low functional health literacy skills, exacerbated by the devastating impacts of poverty and social exclusion, have a real and negative impact on health" (Chapter 8, p. 161). They suggest that some of these inequities could be reduced through addressing dysfunctional practitioner–patient communication. In addition, they suggest that a public health approach connected to health promotion and life-long learning and providing skills and resources to take control of adverse circumstances, particularly though community development, "should reduce inequalities by empowering individuals and communities currently marginalized and at higher risk of developing long-term conditions." (Chapter 8, p. 162).

CREATING BRIDGES WITH OTHERS

There are no doubt other areas of agreement among the authors of this book and likely among the participants in the conference, such as the importance of power as well as policy; but the examples that I have given certainly suggest there are areas of growing consensus among people working in health literacy in different parts of the world as reflected in this book. This is not to suggest that there are no areas of disagreement among them; that certainly is not the case as is implied by the use of the term *perspectives* in the title as well as in its contents. However, perhaps there is enough agreement to move forward toward creating some bridges with others working in health literacy or other fields.

A good example would be the possibility of creating bridges with decision makers, as discussed by Coughlan in Chapter 7. Moreover, he demonstrates how this might be achieved though the questions that we could ask regarding the skills or abilities of individuals and about the demands and complexities of health care system as well as by health literacy advocates understanding the economic data requirements for decision making. In other words, by understanding needs and language of decision makers and speaking with them using this understanding and language, it is possible to create bridges that will help achieve the goals of both the advocates and the decision makers.

Another group that it is possible to create bridges with are researchers who may have somewhat different perspectives from the ones who participated in the conference that produced this book. For example, by coincidence, while working on this Foreword, I received a copy of a large document that emerged from another conference on health literacy that also took place in 2010. That document, published as a supplement by the *Journal of Health Communication,* contains a large number of papers presented at the *Health Literacy Annual Research Conference* held in Washington, DC, in October 2010 as well as editorial materials and two commentaries. Both the conference and the publication differ in a number of ways from the conference and book that I have commented on so far. Specifically, almost all of the authors (and probably conference attendees) were from the United States; only one article had authors from more than one country; there was very little discussion of definitions, context, or the life course; and the majority of articles focused on skills or behaviours of the public, mostly in health care settings. In addition, the overriding focus of the publication was on research, which was in its title. Nevertheless, there are a number of commonalities between the two publications.

Perhaps most notable was one of the two commentaries on measurement in health literacy. It cited a survey of members of a Health Literacy Discussion List that found the following three assertions among the strongest in the responses:

1) New measures of health literacy need to be based on sound theory.
2) Researchers and practitioners need to be able to measure … the health literacy of individuals and the health literacy of health systems and health professionals.
3) A measure of health literacy must allow comparison across contexts including culture, life course, population group, and research setting. (Pleasant, McKinney, & Rikard, 2011, p. 12)

It is interesting to note that the last two points are very similar to some of the previously mentioned points of agreement. In addition, Pleasant et al. provided a long list of limitations of existing measures of health literacy, which certainly is consistent with the consensus among the authors of this book. They also suggested that new measures of health literacy should be based on the same theory or conceptual framework of health literacy, which implies the need for rigorous discussion and analysis of definitions, as suggested in this book. Finally, Pleasant et al. outlined desirable attributes of a comprehensive approach to measuring health literacy, most of which probably would be acceptable to the authors of this book. Thus, their commentary is certainly compatible with this book and, in fact, complements the discussion about measurement by identifying the principles that need to be applied in developing a comprehensive approach.

Other parts of the supplement are also compatible with this book. For example, Ruffin (2011) in the Foreword focused on the elimination of health disparities, another term for health inequalities, and noted the importance of empowerment and culture. Similarly, McCormack, Rush, Kandula, and Paasche-Orlow (2011) in their Introduction to the supplement, mentioned "conceptual disagreements about health literacy" and the need for "clarity and consensus" (p. 7); and in the second commentary, Johnson, Baur, and Meissner (2011) noted the need to "build[...] the bridge between basic and applied research" (p. 28).

In addition, some of the supplement authors presented materials relevant to furthering the discussion and development of some of the issues raised in this book. For example, Pizur-Barnekow, Durragh, and Johnston (2011) presented the findings of a focus group with caregivers of children with medical needs to "better understand the interactive and critical health literacy skills caregivers use when coordinating their children's care." (p. 205), which they suggest may be useful in measuring these types of literacy as well as identifying foci for relevant interventions. Similarly, Macabasco-O'Connell and Fry-Bowers (2011) reported on a pilot study "to describe nursing professionals' knowledge and perceptions of the impact of limited health literacy on individual patients, their practice, and the health system." (p. 298).

Thus, there clearly is an opportunity for creating a bridge between the authors of this book and the authors of the supplement as well as the organizers of the two conferences. In addition, there are other bridges that need to be created. For example, it is noteworthy that none of the authors of either publication were from developing countries. Given that the most recent World Health Organization Health Promotion Conference focused on health literacy, particularly in relation to developing countries, and that the International Union for Health Promotion and Education is in the process of developing a Working Group on Health Literacy, there are opportunities for developing bridges with such countries.

CONCLUSION

It is impossible to do full justice to a book as rich as this one in a 2,500-word Foreword. However, I hope that I have inspired some of you to acquire this book and others to read it. It is well worth the cost and the effort. I also hope that this results in more health literacy bridges being created.

REFERENCES

Johnson, S. E., Baur, C., & Meissner, H. I. (2011). Back to basics: Why basic research is needed to create effective health literacy interventions. *Journal of Health Communication, 16*(Suppl.3), 22-29.

Macabasco-O'Connell, A., & Fry-Bowers, E. K. (2011). Knowledge and perceptions of health literacy among nursing professionals. *Journal of Health Communication, 16*(Suppl.3), 295-307.

McCormack, L. A., Rush, S. R., Kandula, N. R., & Paasche-Orlow, M. K. (2011). Health literacy research: Looking forward. *Journal of Health Communication, 16*(Suppl.3), 5-8.

Pizur-Barnekow, K., Durragh, A., & Johnston, M. (2011). "I cried because I didn't know if I could take care of him": Toward a taxonomy of interactive and critical health literacy as portrayed by caregivers of children with special health care needs. *Journal of Health Communication, 16*(Suppl.3), 205-221.

Pleasant, A., McKinney, J., & Rikard, R. V. (2011). Health literacy measurement: A proposed research agenda. *Journal of Health Communication, 16*(Suppl.3), 11-21.

Ruffin, J. (2011). Foreword: Health literacy and the elimination of health disparities. *Journal of Health Communication, 16*(Suppl.3), 1-2.

Tones, K. (2002). Health literacy: New wine in old bottles? *Health Education Research, 17*, 287-290.

Wister, A. V., Malloy-Weir, L., Rootman, I., & Desjardins, R. (2010). Lifelong educational practices and resources enabling health literacy among older adults. *Journal of Aging and Health, 22*(6), 827-854.

In: Health Literacy in Context   ISBN: 978-1-61942-921-5
Eds.: D.Begoray, D.Gillis, G.Rowlands © 2012 Nova Science Publishers, Inc.

Chapter 1

INTRODUCING HEALTH LITERACY IN CONTEXT

Doris E. Gillis[*], Deborah L. Begoray and Gillian Rowlands

ABSTRACT

Health literacy is an important concept—one that this book considers in context and from different international perspectives. In this chapter, we introduce readers to the evolving concept of health literacy and present a timeline of key events from the first recorded mention of health literacy to the present. In addition, we look at health literacy as both an individual and systemic concern, with some scholars considering it from a clinical point of view and others from a public health or community empowerment view. The health literacy experts from the United States, the United Kingdom, Canada, China, Ireland, and Israel who presented at *Health Literacy: Making the Most of Health* conference that took place in London, England, in February 2010 later wrote the chapters that appear in this book. These chapters are on timely topics relevant to health literacy including definitions, healthy lifestyle, health outcomes, lifelong learning, culture and community, and economics.

[*] Corresponding author: Email: dgillis@stfx.ca.

INTRODUCTION

As citizens of the 21st century, we are expected to understand and use an unprecedented amount and variety of health information from diverse sources. It is within this contemporary challenge that the concept of *health literacy* has emerged as an important topic. Never before has so much attention been directed to health literacy—a concept that is not only capturing the interest of researchers but also inviting health practitioners and policy makers to look at their work in new ways. Health literacy is increasingly referred to as a vital resource for everyday living, a key determinant of health, and a critical aspect of health disparities.

In describing this emerging and multidisciplinary field of research, Paasche-Orlow, McCaffery, and Wolf (2009) claimed that "health literacy has become an international phenomenon" (p. 293). The complexity of health literacy as a construct reflects its international relevance in multiple arenas including health, education, economics, and policy. While those integrating notions of health literacy into their work learn about practices from one another around the world, they must be cognizant that practices are neither neutral nor universally applicable. A consideration for context is vital to the success of health literacy interventions. *Health Literacy in Context: International Perspectives* engages with this complexity. There have been a number of important events in the history of health literacy (Table 1) that may assist readers in putting this book in a chronological context.

HEALTH LITERACY AS BOTH AN INDIVIDUAL AND A SYSTEMIC CONCERN

Health literacy concerns the ways in which people engage with information for their health. It does not refer only to the ability and responsibility of individuals (e.g., as patients, consumers, or citizens) to become more health literate but also to the ability and responsibility of systems through which information relevant to health is provided. Health literacy, therefore, should be a key concern of the practitioners and policy makers within those systems—both inside and outside of health care. Ideally, both individuals and systems must improve and become more health literate.

Table 1. A Timeline of Key Events in the Emergence of Health Literacy

1970s	First reported use of the term 'health literacy' (Simonds, 1974).
1980s	First national literacy surveys showing low levels of basic skills in some population segments. In the United States, physician interest in functional skills and health emerges, leading to multiple studies testing patient literacy and improving readability of health information.
1990s	Canadian Public Health Association takes up the issue of 'literacy and health' and develops plain-language health resources.
1993	Australian policy report defines health literacy as accessing, understanding, and using information to promote and maintain good health (Nutbeam and Wise, 1993).
1994	First international literacy and skills survey (IALS now IALSS).
1998	World Health Organisation (WHO, 1998) definition of health literacy: "Health literacy represents the cognitive and social skills that determine the motivation and ability of individuals to gain access to, understand and use information in ways which promote and maintain good health. Health literacy means more than being able to read pamphlets and successfully make appointments. By improving peoples' access to health information, and their capacity to use it effectively, health literacy is critical to empowerment" (p.10)
1999	First discussion of the 'functional, interactive, and critical health literacy' typology: "Basic/functional literacy: sufficient basic skills in reading and writing to be able to function effectively in everyday situations ... "Communicative/interactive literacy: more advanced cognitive and literacy skills, which together with social skills, can be used to actively participate in everyday activities, to extract information and derive meaning from different forms of communication, and to apply new information to changing circumstances. "Critical literacy: more advanced cognitive skills which, together with social skills, can be applied to critically analyse information, and to use this information to exert greater control over life events and situations." (Nutbeam, 1999; 2000, pp. 263-264)
2002	Health literacy identified in the US *Healthy People 2010* (US Department of Health and Human Services, 2000). "The degree to which individuals have the capacity to obtain, process, and understand basic health information and services needed to make appropriate health decisions" (p. 5).
2003	England's *Skills for Life* adult literacy survey shows low levels of general literacy and numeracy.
2003	*Skilled for Health* adult learning program begins in England.

Table 1. (Continued)

2004	US Institute of Medicine's *Health Literacy: A Prescription to End Confusion* (Nielsen-Bohlman, Panzer, and Kindig, 2004) suggests that "Health literacy goes beyond the individual. It also depends upon the skills, preferences, and expectations of those health information providers: our doctors, nurses, administrators, home health workers, the media, and many others. Health literacy arises from a convergence of education, health services, and social and cultural factors, and brings together research and practice from diverse fields." (p. 2).
2004	The United Kingdom's National Consumer Council releases *Health Literacy: Being Able to Make the Most of Health* (Sihota and Lennard, 2004), which points to "a need to develop a broader-based investigation that goes beyond medically determined studies to include sociological research." (p. 7).
2008	Canadian Expert Panel on Health Literacy reports health literacy as a serious issue and presents a Canadian definition: "The ability to access understand, evaluate and communicate information as a way to promote, maintain and improve health in a variety of settings across the life course" (Rootman and Gordon-El-Bihbety, 2008, p.11).
2010	Conference in London, England on *Health Literacy: Making the Most of Health* brings together international presenters and participants.

It is within this broad understanding of health literacy that this book has been written. In essence, health-literate individuals are able to find, understand, evaluate, and communicate and have the potential to use information to make health decisions throughout the changing circumstances of their lives. Health-literate professionals, service providers, and systems are able to provide relevant information to people in ways that improve their understanding and their capacity to be healthy and to effectively manage their health concerns.

The importance of looking at health literacy as an attribute of both potential users and providers of information was emphasized by the US Institute of Medicine's landmark document, *Health Literacy: A Prescription to End Confusion*: "Health literacy emerges when the expectations, preferences, and skills of individuals seeking health information and services meet the expectations, preferences, and skills of those providing information and services" (Nielsen-Bohlman et al., 2004, p. 2). Creators of more health-literate systems are able to recognize and break down barriers that prevent people from accessing and understanding information and services provided to support health, thus encouraging a better 'fit' between individuals and the systems they use. Thus, health literacy is framed as a "mediator between individuals and the health context" (p. 32). In this book, we explore the many contexts of this interaction in order to gain a better understanding of the evolving concept of health literacy.

HEALTH LITERACY AS A CONCEPT IN FLUX

The concept of health literacy is rooted in understandings of two important concepts: health and literacy—concepts that themselves lack universally shared definitions. Much of the inconsistency in defining health literacy stems from varying perspectives on both health and literacy.

Increasingly, health is defined as a resource for everyday life, not the object of living. According to the 1948 WHO constitution, it is a state of complete physical, mental, and social well-being—not merely the absence of disease or infirmity. This understanding of health places emphasis on social and personal resources as well as physical capabilities (WHO, 1998). Today, health is known to be significantly influenced by a broad range of social determinants (WHO Commission on Social Determinants of Health, 2008). The acknowledgement of the impact and interrelationship of social, economic, political, and environmental conditions on people's capacity to promote and manage their own health, and that of their family and community, highlights concerns about equity and health disparities. Viewing health as "the capacity of people to adapt to, respond to, or control life's challenges and changes" (Frankish, Green, Ratner, Chomik, and Larsen, 1996, Health section, para. 3) is consistent with thinking of health literacy as an important asset for promoting, maintaining, and managing health (Nutbeam, 2008).

Likewise, literacy is a concept that is in flux. Narrow definitions of literacy as only reading and writing, often to some predetermined grade level, have been largely supplanted by notions of multiple literacies that include the ability to read and write, to speak and listen, and to create and understand visuals and multimedia. These communicative abilities are needed for electronically mediated contexts such as those of social media, email, and web searching. All uses of language and literacy are situated in particular times and places (Barton, Hamilton, and Ivanic, 2000), an idea that has significance when considering the multiple circumstances and varied settings in which individuals interact with information that has a bearing on their health.

Although currently no one theory of health literacy exists, many definitions of health literacy have emerged that speak to the various contexts in which health literacy is seen as pertinent (Baker, 2006; Nutbeam, 2008; Pleasant and Kuruvilla, 2008) and that reflect in varying degrees the range of definitions of health and literacy. Health literacy, in turn, has sparked lively debate in the literature reflecting multiple perspectives and approaches of researchers, practitioners, and policy makers. Readers of this book should expect authors to draw from different definitions of health literacy; readers are invited to identify and explore the various ways in which health literacy is conceptualized and operationalized through the examples of practice and policy interventions. In each chapter, these scholars integrate aspects of health literacy into a variety of clinical, health promotion, education, and social practice contexts. In doing so, they identify the challenges confronted in application and the tensions of health literacy as an evolving concept.

AIMS OF THE BOOK

The aims of *Health Literacy in Context: International Perspectives* are several. First, we want to honour the differences in the health literacy concept and then to examine closely the various topics that are currently under investigation by researchers, practitioners, and policy makers involved in health literacy. Our central focus is on the *context* of these comments. By emphasizing context, we mean to invoke the various settings and circumstances in which people (both potential users and providers) interact with information that has relevance to health. Authors discuss understandings and applications of health literacy in a wide range of physical, social, and cultural contexts as they address health issues faced by various populations and across the life course.

Finally, our aim is to engage readers in the consideration of health literacy's implications for health decision making within the context of health care settings as well as the many other settings in which people make choices about their daily lifestyle practices. While some authors frame health literacy as a clinical concern, others view it as a public health or community empowerment priority. For some, it is an issue of improving the health literacy of patients, individuals, and health services; for others, it is about developing a coherent policy or intervention to develop a health-literate society. That health literacy can be looked at in such varied contexts makes it a topic of broad interest and lively debate, which we hope readers will discover for themselves as they read the chapters that follow.

INTERNATIONAL AND INTERDISCIPLINARY PERSPECTIVES OF THE BOOK

Although there is growing evidence substantiating the significant impact of low health literacy on the health and well-being of populations in many countries, many of the developments to date have taken place within, rather than between, disciplinary arenas and international boundaries. This book attempts to bridge that gap. For the first time in one book, international experts from clinical medicine, public health, health promotion, lifelong learning, economics, and public policy present their views on health literacy from their disciplinary perspective. The editors of this book have entered the health literacy arena from different disciplines, drawing upon their experience in the fields of health and literacy and upon their application of biomedical, public health, health promotion, sociology, education, and adult education approaches. A similar variety of backgrounds is found in the authors of this book (For further biographical details, please see pp. 169).

ORIGINS AND ORGANIZATION OF THE BOOK

This edited book evolved from a seminar series of presentations by health literacy experts from the United Kingdom (UK), the United States (US), Canada (CA), China (CN), Ireland (IE), and Israel (IL) that took place in London, England, in February 2010. The idea for this seminar series emerged from the discussions of practitioners and academics in the UK where health literacy as a focus of research, policy, and practice was still in its infancy; however, extensive research and experience had already taken place in other countries and settings. The objective of the conference was to bring together international experts from various disciplines, facilitating both sharing of current knowledge and generation of interdisciplinary discussions that would then enable individuals and organizations to decide upon, and implement, initiatives in their own setting.

Since that time, presenters have continued their dialogue as they updated and prepared chapters. Their chapters reflect this interaction and demonstrate the knowledge and passion they bring to the topic of health literacy. Building on current research and their expertise, authors explore the multifaceted concept of health literacy as it relates to health and wellness, lifestyle decision making, and lifelong learning. The discussion extends beyond an understanding of the health literacy of individuals as potential users of information to examine the health literacy challenges of communities and the wider social, cultural, and economic relevance of health literacy.

This book is timely in that each chapter provides a synthesis of current knowledge with identification of gaps and perspectives on the conceptualization and operationalization of health literacy. Authors make reference to ongoing research pertaining, for example, to the development of measurement tools, innovative approaches to practice, evaluation of interventions, and, where applicable, the policy implications arising from the work they describe. Authors also suggest directions for future research.

Health Literacy in Context: International Perspectives offers *Questions for Reflection* at the end of each chapter. Readers can use these prompts as ways to move their own thinking forward. Educators might consider the questions as topics for small- or large-group discussion and journal or essay prompts for writing. These questions are posed in an effort to further the conversation on health literacy begun in London in 2010, in particular, to consider implications of this important concept for rethinking current practice, advancing policy development, and increasing understanding through future research.

In addition, there is an *Index* at the end of this book to assist readers in finding topics of particular interest.

OVERVIEW OF HEALTH LITERACY IN CONTEXT: INTERNATIONAL PERSPECTIVES

In the Foreword, *Creating Bridges with Health Literacy*, Irv Rootman (CA) provides commentary that links the various health literacy topics and themes of this book from his perspective as a researcher and health literacy advocate.

In Chapter 1, the Editors offer readers an introduction to the content and debates of health literacy pursued within this book and give readers an overview of its structure.

In Chapter 2 *Health Literacy and Definitions of Terms*, Rima Rudd (US), Alexa McCray (US), and Donald Nutbeam (UK) address the evolution of health literacy as a concept, including shifts in its usage over time and the tools developed to measure it. These authors describe how health literacy has emerged from the study of the links between education and health. They discuss selected definitions of health literacy and how these result in different approaches to researching and understanding the associations among health literacy and health and well-being. They describe how differing definitions focus either on the skills of individuals or on the design of health systems. The chapter ends with a call to widen the field of health literacy research to include more attention on context, including the facilitators and barriers influencing people's access and engagement with health information. The authors also call for further development of appropriate ways to take into account contextual characteristics in evaluating health literacy interventions.

In Chapter 3 *Health Literacy and Healthy Lifestyle Choices,* Doris Gillis (CA) and Nicola Gray (UK) examine health literacy and healthy lifestyle choices within the current debate about the relative focus of individual responsibility for healthy lifestyle behaviour versus social responsibility through public policy addressing the social determinants of health. Drawing on two examples, England and Canada, they examine policy discourse that situates health literacy as it pertains to the promotion of healthy lifestyles. These authors present two case studies drawn from their respective professions of nutrition and pharmacy to examine how dimensions of health literacy are reflected in practice. In so doing, they identify tensions embedded in the notion of informed choice as it relates to promoting healthy lifestyle practices.

In Chapter 4 *Health Literacy and Health Outcomes,* Joanne Protheroe (UK), Michael Wolf (US), and Albert Lee (CN) propose that lifestyle choices and behaviours, combined with the environments where people live and work and genetic susceptibility, lead to measurable associations between health literacy and health. This chapter reviews the body of research exploring associations between adult literacy skills and health outcomes. General literacy and health literacy have been linked to problems with the use of preventive services, delayed diagnoses, understanding of one's medical condition, adherence to medical instructions, self-management skills, physical and mental health, and increased mortality. The nature of these relationships are examined in detail and likely causal pathways discussed.

In Chapter 5 *Health Literacy and Lifelong Learning,* Deborah Begoray (CA), Anne Marshall (CA), Laura Shone (US), and Gillian Rowlands (UK) describe how health literacy, by its very nature, straddles the health and education domains. Whereas the preceding two chapters viewed health literacy from a health perspective, this chapter views health literacy through the education or lifelong learning lens. Health and health literacy, then, can be excellent topics around which to develop general literacy and numeracy skills. Conversely, there is extensive evidence that developing skills, in whatever area, leads to better health and well-being. This chapter outlines the importance of physical, mental, emotional, and spiritual health to the continuing positive development of individuals and communities and, more specifically, the importance of health literacy and mental health literacy at every stage of life. As an example of good practice, this chapter describes *Skills for Health*, a UK program that combines health and literacy learning. The authors examine this program specifically for various elements of health literacy and lifelong learning.

In Chapter 6 *Health Literacy, Culture, and Community*, Diane Levin-Zamir (IL) and Jane Wills (UK) argue that people are more than just individuals; they are part of communities. As such, an understanding of culture is central to efforts to advance health literacy especially in marginalized groups. These authors discuss the health literacy challenges of specific groups within communities including older adults, migrants, and immigrants and cultures in transition from traditional to western societies. They also consider implications of virtual communities on health literacy. Using case studies from the UK and Israel, they demonstrate that applying the concept of health literacy can go beyond literacy and numeracy to building capacity for health through supporting advocacy skills and empowerment. These authors identify key knowledge gaps that could be addressed by future research addressing health literacy in the community context.

In Chapter 7 *Health Literacy: An Economic Perspective*, Diarmuid Coughlan (IE) argues that the economic data requirements for decision making must be understood by health literacy advocates. He examines important questions about health literacy related to the skills/abilities of individuals and to the demands/complexities of the health care system. On the one side, he asks: Are health-literate individuals more efficient users of health care resources? Can we produce better health through investing in health literacy? Do health literacy interventions improve one's health outcomes? On the demand/complexity side, he asks: How does a third-party investor view health literacy? What incentive is there for a provider to advocate health literacy principles? How should policy makers approach health literacy? A case study in England is used to support Coughlan's discussion.

Chapter 8 *Concluding Thoughts and the Future of Health Literacy*, features the Editors drawing together threads from the preceding chapters, highlighting the key themes and messages relevant to current knowledge about health literacy, and offering emerging insights on policy implications. Finally, predictions are offered for the future of health literacy based on signposts from events in the history of health literacy found earlier in this chapter.

AN INVITATION TO READERS

This book takes readers through a rich discussion of what is meant by the term *health literacy* and how health literacy is important in multiple contexts. It will be of particular appeal to practitioners, students, and educators at both undergraduate and graduate levels interested in learning more about the interplay of health literacy and the complex set of determinants of health. Today's health and social professionals, and those involved in their education, are called upon to integrate health literacy into practice within a wide range of contexts and settings and through various disciplines and roles. We, the editors, hope that practitioners, policy makers, and researchers will find value in the multiple disciplinary and international perspectives on health literacy presented, the examples of innovative practice given, and the identification of gaps in knowledge and directions for future research suggested.

REFERENCES

Baker, D. W. (2006). The meaning and measure of health literacy. *Journal of General Internal Medicine*, *21*(8), 878-883. doi:10.1111/j.1525-1497.2006.00540.x.

Barton, N. D., Hamilton, M., and Ivanic, R. (Eds.). (2000). *Situated literacies: Reading and writing in context.* London, England: Routledge.

Frankish, C. J., Green, L. W., Ratner, P. A., Chomik, T., and Larsen, C. (1996). *Health impact assessment as a tool for population health promotion and public policy* (Report to the Health Promotion Development Division of Health Canada). Vancouver, Canada: Institute of Health Promotion Research, University of British Columbia. Retrieved from http://www.phac-aspc.gc.ca/ph-sp/impact-repercussions/.

Nielsen-Bohlman, L., Panzer, A.M., and Kindig, D. A. (2004). *Health literacy: A prescription to end confusion.* Committee on Health Literacy, Board on Neuroscience and Behavioral Health, Institute of Medicine. Washington, DC: The National Academies Press.

Nutbeam, D. (1999). Literacies across the lifespan: Health literacy. *Literacy and Numeracy Studies, 9*(2), 47-55.

Nutbeam, D. (2000). Health literacy as a public health goal: A challenge for contemporary health education and communication strategies into the 21st century. *Health Promotion International, 15*(3), 259-267.

Nutbeam, D. (2008). The evolving concept of health literacy. *Social Science and Medicine, 67*(12), 2072-2078.

Nutbeam, D., and Wise, M. (1993). Australia: Planning for better health. *Promotion and Education,* 19-24.

Paasche-Orlow, M. K., McCaffery, K., and Wolf, M. S. (2009). Bridging the international divide for health literacy research. *Patient Education and Counseling, 75,* 293-294.

Pleasant, A., and Kuruvilla, S. (2008). A tale of two health literacies: Public health and clinical approaches to health literacy. *Health Promotion International, 23*(2), 152-159.

Rootman, I., and Gordon-El-Bihbety, D. (2008). *A vision for a health literate Canada: Report of the expert panel on health literacy.* Ottawa, Canada: Canadian Public Health Association.

Sihota, S., and Lennard, L. (2004). *Health literacy: Being able to make the most of health.* London, England: National Consumer Council.

Simonds, S. K. (1974). Health education as social policy. *Health Education Monograph 2,* 1-25.

United States Department of Health and Human Services. (2000). *Healthy people 2010: Understanding and improving health.* Washington, DC: Author.

World Health Organization. (1998). *Health promotion glossary.* Geneva, Switzerland: Author.

World Health Organization. (2008). *Closing the gap in a generation: Health equity through action on the social determinants of health.* Geneva, Switzerland: World Health Organization Commission on Social Determinants of Health.

In: Health Literacy in Context   ISBN: 978-1-61942-921-5
Eds.: D.Begoray, D.Gillis, G.Rowlands   © 2012 Nova Science Publishers, Inc.

Chapter 2

HEALTH LITERACY AND DEFINITION OF TERMS

Rima E. Rudd[*], *Alexa T. McCray*
and Donald Nutbeam

ABSTRACT

In recent years, health literacy has emerged as a substantive and rich field of inquiry. However, there has not always been full agreement on what exactly is meant by the term *health literacy* itself. With health literacy increasingly considered a social determinant of health, focused attention to its definition is warranted. A definition not only sets parameters but also indirectly shapes questions for inquiry; it offers guidelines for measurement and, in the case of health literacy, indicates a locus of control and responsibility that may influence research, practice, and policy decisions. Early definitions of health literacy focused on the skills and abilities of individuals to gain access to, understand, and use information. However, attention has been increasingly focused on the assumptions and skills of those professionals who develop and provide health messages, directions, and information and on those institutions providing services and care. This growing attention to the physical and social contexts of health activities calls for renewed attention to the definition of health literacy with its focus on individuals. We argue that a more comprehensive definition of health literacy must include both the

---

[*] Corresponding author: E-mail: rrudd@hsph.harvard.edu.

abilities of individuals and the characteristics of professionals and institutions that support or that may inhibit individual or community action. Any such definition will unquestionably need to be accompanied by measurement tools that fully operationalize its key concepts—thereby including not only measurements of the abilities of the lay public but also of the texts, of the skills of health professionals, and of the expectations and assumptions of health care environments.

INTRODUCTION

Links between education and health outcomes have been well established. Only recently, however, has literacy—the foundation stone of education—been examined as a pathway to health. This interest in the links between literacy and health has garnered a good deal of attention from researchers, practitioners, and policy makers over the past decade and has established health literacy as a substantive field of inquiry. Contributions to the field include over 1,500 peer-reviewed articles in health journals, several texts, multiple editorials, white papers, and policy reports (Berkman, Sheridan, Donohue, Halpern, and Crotty, 2011; Rudd, Anderson, Oppenheimer, and Nath, 2007).

At the same time, defining *health literacy* has been somewhat problematic, causing many contributors to the field to pose and then revisit those definitions. Without a commonly agreed-upon definition, there is little or no control over words. Indeed, a term may be so broadly defined or so narrowly applied that misconceptions and misunderstandings result. In addition, it may be so variously defined that each usage requires a precise delineation so that communication can proceed.

> 'When I use a word,' Humpty Dumpty said, in a rather scornful tone, 'it means just what I choose it to mean – neither more nor less.' (Carroll, 1871)

It is difficult, in scholarly discourse or public engagement, to have the kind of personal control that Humpty Dumpty sought over the use of words. Consequently, definitions help maintain clarity. A definition not only sets parameters but also indirectly shapes questions for inquiry; it offers guidelines for measurement and, in the case of health literacy, indicates a locus of control and responsibility that may influence practice and policy decisions. In this chapter, we focus on the definitions and uses of the term *health literacy* with attention to shifts in usage over time as well as to the tools developed to measure health literacy.

IMPORTANCE OF TERMS

With health literacy increasingly considered a social determinant of health, focused attention to the construct is warranted. Scholars and practitioners newly engaged in shaping a health literacy agenda within their area of work and will want to closely examine the concepts and underlying assumptions that have shaped and are shaping health literacy work elsewhere. Of on-going interest is attention to the title itself and to the meaning and implications of terms used.

Research protocols demand that key terms be carefully defined and operationalized. Indeed, construct validity is determined by the extent to which the constructs are successfully measured. Consequently, attention to definitions of terms must include a discussion of measures. In addition, definitions hold importance beyond individual studies because they may influence a field by establishing parameters on the focus and scope of inquiry. Thus, this chapter offers an overview of definitions and measures with an understanding that definitions have consequences for the rigor of individual studies as well as for a field as a whole.

In general, definitions are biased and, when closely examined, yield insight into a particular perspective. Bias is understood to be a predisposed tendency toward a certain point of view, which is most often based on a particular system of beliefs including orientation, personal knowledge, and experience. The term *bias* is not used to imply incorrect or nonsensical definitions. We do note, however, that underlying beliefs and perspectives need to be recognized and their consequences need to be addressed (McCray, 2006). Thus, we intend that the discussion provided in this chapter sets the foundation for an examination of key questions related to health literacy research: What constitutes health literacy? How will it be measured? Who and what will be measured?

BACKGROUND

Studies focused on the relationship between health and literacy began, of course, with literacy. Definitions and measures of *literacy* vary widely—including, for example, the ability to sign one's name, the ability to read proffered text aloud, the proof of having attended school, the acquisition of a high school diploma. Generally, literacy is understood to have two distinctive elements: those that are task-based and those that are skills-based. Task-based literacy focuses on the extent to which a person can perform key literacy tasks, such as read a basic text and write a simple statement. Skills-based literacy focuses on the knowledge and skills an adult must possess in order to perform these tasks. These skills range from basic, word-level skills (e.g., recognizing words) to higher-level skills (e.g., drawing appropriate inferences from continuous text). Importantly, it follows that literacy can be measured in absolute terms by distinguishing between those who can read and write basic text and those who cannot and in relative terms as well by assessing the skill differences between those who are able to perform relatively challenging literacy tasks and those who are not.

In the late 1980s, a group of education scholars developed a uniform measure of literacy that could be used by industrialized nations for national and for comparative international analyses. They did so by assembling and analyzing commonly available materials (e.g., newspaper and magazine articles, bank deposit slips, bus schedules, merchandise labels) from various aspects of everyday life (e.g., finance, civics, work, health, recreation) and then evaluating them in terms of complexity. Materials were divided into prose (continuous text such as an editorial or health pamphlet) and documents (e.g., lists, charts, graphs) and ranged from simple to complex. Tasks were developed to resemble those most likely undertaken for everyday activities and were ranked by level of difficulty. For example, a survey participant might be asked to determine the winning team, using a sports article on a recent game (i.e., locate one piece of information in an article without distractions). A participant, given a common over-the-counter medicine box, would be asked to use the information to decide how much medicine to give a child of a specified age and weight (i.e., use a complex chart to find multiple pieces of information). Another may be asked to identify the writer's perspective in a newspaper editorial (i.e., interpret text to identify implicit opinions). Thus, the survey examined functional literacy based on materials and specific tasks related to them (Kirsch, 2001). These assessments were based on an agreed-upon measure of literacy as a functional skill—the ability to use commonly available materials to accomplish mundane tasks.

Findings from the 1992 United States (US) National Adult Literacy Survey (NALS) and from the International Adult Literacy Surveys (IALS) conducted in 1994 in Canada and 20 other industrialized nations indicated that large proportions of adults had difficulty using print materials to accomplish everyday tasks with accuracy and consistency. Analyses of these surveys and of those that followed in 2003 provided evidence that the literacy skills of a majority of adults in most countries were not adequate to meet the expectations and demands of their societies (Kirsch, Jungeblut, Jenkins, and Kolstad, 1993; Kutner, Greenberg, and Baer, 2005; Murray, Kirsch, and Jenkins, 1997). Furthermore, differences in literacy proficiency based on educational attainment, poverty, and access to resources and on majority versus minority status indicated powerful effects of social factors (Rudd, 2007; Rudd, Kirsch, and Yamamoto, 2004). Analysts determined that literacy attainment is influenced by a variety of social factors and, in turn, that literacy skills further determine opportunities, employment, and social engagement (Sum, Kirsch, and Taggart, 2002). These insights set a foundation for examinations of literacy as a contributor to health outcomes and as a mediating factor in health disparities.

Literacy and Health

Before the NALS and IALS surveys were undertaken, Grosse and Auffrey (1989) had traced the development of research on literacy as a major determinant of health status to studies in developing nations. Their public health review article helped establish the now-acknowledged links between maternal literacy and the health of children. Soon thereafter, published findings of international assessments of adult literacy skills drew the attention of health researchers and practitioners working in industrialized nations. The primary questions for these research initiatives focused on the health implications of the documented literacy skills of adults.

After publication of the educational survey findings in the early 1990s, literacy and its implications for health outcomes and disparities became the focus of a growing number of health studies in several English-speaking countries. Interest in health and literacy emerged as a policy issue in Canada and in Australia in the early 1990s (Nutbeam and Wise, 1993; Rootman and Gordon-El-Bihbety, 2008). Research studies were launched in the US soon thereafter. Publications in peer-reviewed journals grew from about 50 during the years 1960–1989 to over 300 by 1999, with over 1,500 publications in the first decade of the 21st century (Rudd et al., 2007; Rudd and Keller, 2009; Rudd, Moeykens, and Colton, 2000).

Health Literacy Research Strands and Tools

Two major strands of research have shaped the field of health literacy. The first focus of study was on the materials and messages developed for consumer use. This area expanded over time to include analyses of materials and messages in print and online, the match between text characteristics and the skills of intended readers, and analyses of spoken messages. Over 1,000 studies now indicate that demands are indeed quite high—above the average skills of a majority of adults—rendering a good deal of health information, if not useless, of limited use (Rudd et al., 2007).

Most of the tools used for studies of health materials and messages focused on only two characteristics of text: word and sentence length. However, this initial and somewhat superficial measure offered insight into challenges people face as they try to decode health information and supported arguments for examining and refining commonly used materials. Several workbooks and texts, such as Doak, Doak, and Root's classic text *Teaching Patients with Low Literacy Skills* (1996), helped people move beyond attention to word and sentence length to examine writing style as well as organizational and design elements that ease or hinder the reading process. Subsequent developments included attention to document format (Mosenthal and Kirsch, 1998), web posting (Choi and Bakken, 2010; Friedman and Hoffman-Goetz, 2006), and numeracy demands in health care settings (Apter et al., 2008).

The second strand of research focused on the links between literacy skills of individuals and a variety of health-related outcomes. In the mid 1990s, health researchers in the US were inspired by findings from the 1992 NALS to develop measurement tools that could be administered in health settings and used in research inquiries to examine health-related differences between patients with strong literacy skills and patients with weak literacy skills. The resulting tools were approximations of reading skills based on health-related words or statements from commonly used materials. They were modified over time as developers responded to preference for instruments that could be administered quickly within medical settings (Davis et al., 1993; Parker, Baker, Williams, and Nurss, 1995; Weiss et al., 2005). A continued interest in the development and refinement of measurement tools for health-related fieldwork enabling researchers to assess literacy skills of patients is evident in the development of discipline-specific tools, such as a tool for use in dental research (Lee, Rozier, Lee, Bender, and Ruiz, 2007).

The studies in this strand of research moved from measures of individuals' skills in health contexts to analyses of links between these measured skills and a variety of outcomes including knowledge, behaviours, morbidity, and mortality. Early studies of the links between patients' skills and health outcomes focused on patients in emergency departments and those managing a chronic disease. Over time, health practitioners and clinicians from a broader array of interests (e.g., dentistry, mental health, surgery) have launched studies of patient skills and health outcomes.

By the end of the 1990s, findings from numerous studies indicated an association between reading skills and a variety of health outcomes ranging from knowledge to behaviours. The US federal Agency for Healthcare Research and Quality (AHRQ) commissioned a systematic research review with articulated inclusion criteria. The analytic review weighed the evidence accumulated by 2003 and concluded that the links between literacy skills and health outcomes were well established (DeWalt, Berkman, Sheridan, Lohr, and Pignone, 2004). AHRQ commissioned a second review that found strong links between measured skills and health outcomes (Berkman et al., 2011). The current literature contains dozens of studies concluding that knowledge and understanding of a disease or treatment plan, engagement in preventive behaviours, management of chronic diseases as well as a variety of morbidity and mortality measures vary by literacy skill levels, which were most often estimated through approximations of reading skill.

At the same time, critiques of existing measurement tools highlighted the narrow focus of health literacy studies on the reading skills of patients without attention to other skills, such as speaking, listening, and mathematics (Nielsen-Bohlman, Panzer, and Kindig, 2004). Several recent studies have focused on the importance of dialogue in health, addressing oral and aural literacy (Koch-Weser, Rudd, and DeJong, 2010; Roter, Erby, Larson, and Ellington, 2007, 2009). Two studies examining the relationship between oral literacy and health outcomes measured skills with the Woodcock Johnson Achievements Tests, reported as grade equivalents to explore associations between aural literacy skills and chronic disease management (Rosenfeld, Rudd, Emmons, Acevedo-Garcia, and Buka, 2011) and between reading, numeracy, and aural skills and coronary heart disease risk (Martin et al., 2011). This strand of research, sparked by publication of findings from the adult literacy surveys, has indeed explored the health implications of limited literacy skills. The prevailing definitions of health literacy helped shape this agenda.

Expanding Research and Merging Strands

Much of the literature in this growing area of research has focused on the serious problems that people with low literacy face when interacting with health care systems. This is often viewed, quite appropriately, as a health disparity issue, particularly since those with low literacy have been shown to suffer worse outcomes than those with higher levels of literacy. However, while individuals with low literacy will certainly find it extraordinarily difficult to navigate today's complicated health care system, the US National Academies of Science's Institute of Medicine (IOM) reminds us that even those with strong literacy skills have trouble obtaining, understanding, and using health information (Nielsen-Bohlman et al., 2004). This may mean that we need to look at a very large continuum of needs for those who are at the lowest end of the literacy spectrum to those who are at the highest end, but it may also be the case that an entirely different model is required to understand and address the health literacy needs of otherwise literate individuals.

Furthermore, a substantial portion of the literature on health literacy addresses the problem of the basic literacy level of the patient, the readability of the health-related materials that the patient is expected to read, and the frequent mismatch between the two. However, navigating today's health care system carries with it a high literacy burden. Patients need to interact in a variety of health care settings (e.g., doctors' offices, clinics, hospitals), and they need to interact with a broad range of health-related information (e.g., therapeutic instructions, patient education materials, prescriptions, bills, insurance forms). In addition, they are being asked to take increasingly greater responsibility for their own health care and disease management. Health literacy research has expanded at the same time that health systems have grown increasingly complex (McCray, 2005; Rudd, Renzulli, Perreira, and Daltroy, 2004).

Most of the early definitions of terms and many of the new and expanded definitions continue to draw attention to the skills and capacities of individuals and of communities. However, they do not fully address the capacity of health systems or health professionals to inhibit or enhance such capabilities. While research indicates that the skills of individuals are linked to untoward health outcomes, illness and premature death may well be the result not of the limited literacy skills, capabilities, and desires of the public but instead of a mismatch between the demands of health information and care systems and the literacy skills of population groups (US National Institutes of Health, 2006).

DEFINITIONS OF HEALTH LITERACY

Various definitions of health literacy are found in the literature. This brief history highlights some key documents to discuss both the scope of the definition and the implication for measurement and research.

Capabilities of Individuals

In the US, the National Literacy Act of 1991 was enacted to ensure that all adults in the US acquire basic skills necessary to function effectively and achieve the greatest possible opportunity in their work and in their lives. Literacy was defined as skills needed by adults to function in society, to achieve their goals, and to develop their knowledge and potential (Irwin, 1991). This functional definition of literacy shaped the subsequent assessments of adult literacy skills in industrialized nations and influenced the definitions of health literacy.

Early definitions of health literacy focused on the skills and abilities of individuals to gain access to, understand, and use information. The 1993 Australian policy report defined health literacy in terms of accessing, understanding, and using information to promote and maintain good health (Nutbeam and Wise, 1993). Subsequently, a more expansive definition of health literacy was included in the World Health Organization's (WHO) *Health Promotion Glossary* (1998) written by Nutbeam: "Health literacy represents the cognitive and social skills which determine the motivation and ability of individuals to gain access to, understand and use information in ways which promote and maintain good health." (p. 10).

The glossary section further explains that health literacy means more than reading alone: "Health literacy implies the achievement of a level of knowledge, personal skills and confidence to take action to improve personal and community health by changing personal lifestyles and living conditions." (WHO, 1998, p. 10). Mention of health literacy was included in several other WHO glossary items; it was posited as critical to empowerment and as an important component of participation. In the discussion of participation, health literacy is equated with or linked to health learning: "Health literacy/health learning fosters participation." (WHO, p. 2). Health literacy is also proposed as a measure or outcome, for example, considered useful as a health indicator. Furthermore, the definitions include implicit actions: gain access, understand, use, and participate. However, the term was not operationalized and specific measures were not offered.

The well-articulated connection between health literacy and activation reflected in parts of the WHO health promotion glossary was not overtly incorporated in the burgeoning research in the US. The definition of health literacy used in the US policy document, *Healthy People 2010* (US Department of Health and Human Services [HHS], 2000) focused on individuals' capacities and drew from the previously noted definition of literacy in the 1991 Health Literacy Act. It focuses on individuals' capacity to obtain, process, and understand basic health information and services. This emphasis fits well with the strand of research focused on the capacity/skills of individuals within health care settings but does not quite incorporate attention to the larger arena of health-related action, to the shape and content of the health information, or to the barriers or facilitating factors of available health and health care services.

Health Contexts

In 2003, the HHS action plan for health communication (2003) used the narrowly focused definition generally adopted in its health goals and objectives for the nation but simultaneously highlighted the importance of attending to the assumptions, demands, and skills of those crafting health messages. Similarly, in 2004 the IOM Committee on Health Literacy adopted the same narrow definition with an added caveat that called attention to the importance of both the skill and demand side. The IOM report (Nielsen-Bohlman et al., 2004) called for policy makers to consider the interaction between the skills of individuals and the demands of social systems and to make needed correctives. Baker (2006) proposed a conceptual model that included the complexity and difficulty of print as well as spoken messages and its contribution to the abilities of individuals to understand and communicate. Other researchers have focused attention on the important exchanges taking place in health care settings and explored listening and speaking skills and their influence on chronic disease management as well as for advocacy

(Martin et al., 2011; Rosenfeld et al., 2011; Roter, Erby, Larson, Elllington, 2009).

The 2010 *National Action Plan to Improve Health Literacy* (HHS, 2010) included a broader focus on the demand side by calling for greater skill development to support independence in health decision making and empowerment among individuals and communities and for transformations in health systems to redress the mismatch between current demands and current skills. A responsibility for removing literacy-related barriers has a well-established theoretical foundation in Lewin's force field analysis. According to Lewin (1943), change can best take place when counter-forces are diminished; consequently, before one promotes or encourages action on the part of individuals and communities, one must mitigate or remove existing barriers.

As health literacy researchers became more attentive to the barriers involved in the use of words, jargon phrases, numbers, and numeric concepts, some focused their attention on the skills of health professionals. Several North American medical schools include training related to health literacy (Harper, Cook, and Makloul, 2007). Roter, Erby, Larson, and Ellington (2007, 2009) have encouraged such work by adding health literacy issues to their on-going studies of patient/provider communication. They noted that providers must pay attention to multiple components of communication and interaction (e.g., openings for interruptions, easy flow of exchange, question-asking) in order to shape an encounter that does not presuppose advanced literacy skills. Others have provided initial tools for assessing the literacy environment of health care settings (Groene and Rudd, 2011; Rudd and Anderson, 2006). However, there is still no uniform health literacy tool to assess the skills of providers or institutions. The ability to conduct rigorous research into efficacious change will rely, in part, on the development of sophisticated measures to clearly document and identify existing barriers and to compare and contrast the newly changed environment and so determine change—benefits, deficits, and/or unanticipated outcomes.

At the same time, most individuals may only occasionally be patients. People take action to maintain their health and that of loved ones, fellow workers, members of their community, and their environment. Definitions of health literacy, to be relevant to social and civic engagement, must include attention to action outside of the medical care encounter and broaden the notion of health action to include activities people engage in their homes, communities, and worksites and in the social and political environments of countries and regions (Rudd, 2007). This broader notion (well articulated in the WHO *Health Promotion Glossary*) might include acknowledgement of and attention to the active engagement of lay and professional people as well as institutional action to remove barriers to health-promoting actions. Such an expansion calls for the development of measurement tools so that rigorous program evaluation studies can determine efficacious change.

Expanding Definitions

The discussions of health literacy and proposed definitions of terms in Europe and in Australia, as noted earlier, did not remain static. Instead, health literacy was proposed to be more than the application of literacy skills for finding information and completing health tasks. A typology of health literacy concepts proposed in 2000 transformed existing concepts (Nutbeam, 2000). A newly shaped definition called attention to the application of basic skills but then highlighted the importance of agency and the need to consider the patient/individual as an active participant in the creation of health. The typology included functional, interactive, and critical health literacy. Those working with health literacy at the most basic level—health literacy as functional—tend to focus on access to information and the application of reading skills to enhance understanding and control over events. However, the concept of health literacy as interactive or critical broadens the scope and purview to include active engagement and participation in decision making on individual, community, and policy levels.

This definition, based on an underlying notion of empowerment, has shaped a European concept of health literacy with an emphasis on the individual (i.e., patient or community member) poised to take action. The concept of critical health literacy—the capacity for effective social, political, and individual action—is reflected in the call for recognition of health literacy as an asset and a goal (Nutbeam, 2008). This is reflected in calls in the US for a notion of broader concepts (IOM, 2004; Rudd, 2010). For example, Zarcadoolas, Pleasant, and Greer (2005) proposed a concept of a civic literacy that encompasses the idea of citizens becoming aware of issues, participating in critical dialogue, and becoming involved in decision-making processes for health. Health literacy is defined as "the wide range of skills, and competencies that people develop to seek out, comprehend, evaluate and use health information and concepts to make informed choices, reduce health risks and increase quality of life" (Zarcadoolas, Pleasant and Greer, 2005, p. 196).

Others have proposed variations on definitions that highlight a public health purview. For example, two definitions of public health literacy have been offered. Gazmararian, Curran, Parker, Bernhardt, and DeBuono (2005) suggested that public health literacy enables people to understand the problems of health for themselves, their families, and their communities. Furthermore, they proposed that "a skilled and professional workforce in healthcare and public health will communicate with the public in ways that they understand." (p. 321). Similarly addressing a public health issue, Freedman et al. (2009) suggested that public health literacy engage a broad swath of stakeholders in public health efforts to address social and environmental determinants of health. They proposed that public health literacy is "the degree to which individuals and groups can obtain, process, understand, evaluate, and act upon information needed to make public health decisions that benefit the community" (Freedman et al., 2009, p. 448). Here, different levels of health literacy are distinguished by the higher levels of knowledge and skills that progressively support greater autonomy and personal empowerment in health-related decision making as well as engagement with a wider range of health knowledge. The concept extends from personal health management to the social determinants of health.

Still missing from many of the definitions is one that reflects the active involvement and skills of those in public health and in health care—the administrators, the staff, the writers, the legislators, and the various professionals—who give shape to health information as well as to the physical and social contexts of health activities. A broad concept of health literacy as the capacity for effective social, political, and individual action demands attention to social and political factors that inhibit or support such action.

IMPLICATIONS AND CONCLUSIONS

Literacy assessments in multiple industrialized countries have firmly established weaknesses in the literacy skills of the public. The reason we care so much about literacy is that even the most basic functional literacy skills enable people to better develop their knowledge and improve the potential to achieve personal goals. Thus, they are able to participate more fully in society, both economically and socially. Responding to low levels of literacy in a population involves improving access to effective school education and providing adult literacy programs for those in need. Achieving high levels of literacy in a population is not only a vital development goal; it also produces substantial public health benefits. The documented links between literacy skills and health outcomes call for action.

At the same time, over 1,000 studies indicating a mismatch between health information materials and the documented skills of the general public have firmly established weaknesses in health systems (Nielsen-Bohlman et al., 2004; Rudd and Keller, 2009). If poor communication is at least partially responsible for untoward health and fatalities, swift action is needed to transform the skills of health professionals and the demands of health systems (Rudd, 2010).

Obviously, both groups of action are called for. Currently, we have the measures to track changes in literacy skills and the tools to assess health messages but are missing key measures to study more than basic functional health literacy or to monitor and evaluate efficacious change in health professionals and in health systems. It is far too easy for researchers to apply tools at hand and, perhaps, forget that core components remain undocumented and unmeasured. A definition that will benefit both research and practice should be coupled with measurement tools that can fully operationalize the key concepts.

Unfortunately, many health literacy inquiries—although emphasizing the importance of access to information—tend to focus on and measure the reading skills of individuals and pay scant attention to the characteristics of texts or speech that make information easy to access or too complex for either word recognition or comprehension. Similarly, as the expanding concept of health literacy more regularly includes social, political, and individual action, attention must be given to both the abilities of individuals or communities and the characteristics of institutions and professionals that support or that may inhibit individual or community action. Explorations of how to encourage, support, and establish conducive environments for critical health literacy have not yet been launched, measured, and studied. Certainly, such efforts will include attention to the abilities of health professionals and the capability of health systems to support and actively encourage the capacity for effective social, political, and individual action. Here too, measures of skills of professionals and of environmental characteristics have yet to be fully explored and tested. Until such measures are developed, links between system-level demands and health outcomes cannot be studied.

Furthermore, attention must be given to the logic and underlying assumptions inherent in the new and developing definitions of health literacy. Health literacy studies in the US and several other countries offer a strong research base establishing links between limited literacy skills of individuals and untoward health outcomes. At the same time, we know that literacy does not exist in a vacuum and that measures of skills will show variations based on context and text as well as on unspoken assumptions and demands. Logic cannot support a causal relationship between literacy and health outcomes absent attention to the demand side. Thus, knowledge gaps include the lack of explanatory models that link literacy and social environmental conditions to health outcomes for population groups. Zarcadoolas (2011) proposed that, in taking on a very narrow definition of health literacy, we built a field without a theory.

Health literacy is currently garnering attention in health research, policy, and practice across industrialized nations. A substantial body of research indicates that health materials and other related demands exceed the literacy skills of large numbers of adults in all industrialized nations. Furthermore, a rigorous body of work over the past decade has established a clear link between the reading skills of patients and significant health outcomes. Yet, these two research strands have only recently been connected in a way that supports research into the interplay between skills of individuals and processes within health systems. In part, a narrow definition of health literacy encouraged a myopic focus on literacy deficits of people and ignored the barriers erected by the culture, language, and assumptions of those in the health fields. Only recently have these two research strands been connected in ways that support a critical assessment of the full health literacy environment. Scholars and practitioners will want to closely examine the concepts and underlying assumptions that have shaped health literacy discussion, research, and policy thereby opening the field and the terms in use to more critical scrutiny.

A growing awareness of the importance of definitions and their concurrent measures is encouraging a re-examination of assumptions in the field. Consequently, the highlighted caveats to the prevailing definition of health literacy provided in the early reports from the HHS, *Communicating Health* (2003), and from the IOM, *Health Literacy: A Prescription to End Confusion* (2004), are being revisited in the US; and increased attention is being paid to the more sophisticated notions of health literacy proposed in discussions in Europe. The early focus on the skills of individuals alone is being corrected with increased attention being paid to the health context: the facilitating factors and barriers that support or inhibit access to information and active engagement of people. At the same time, until new and more appropriate measures are developed to measure contextual characteristics and assess engagement, research will be hampered and examinations of possible efficacious action will be stymied.

Questions for Reflection

1) The notion that definitions are inherently biased is introduced at the start of the article. How might the perspectives of varying professionals (e.g., educators, doctors, public health practitioners) influence the definition of health literacy? Which definitions reflect the perspective of which disciplines?

2) Texts in research methods highlight the importance of defining and operationalizing a key concept. How would you define health literacy for each of the two strands of research? How do you judge the adequacy of the measures used?

3) How would you expand the definition of critical health literacy to include attention to the health context/environment?

ACKNOWLEDGMENT

We offer thanks to Lindsay Schubiner SM, graduate research assistant, Harvard School of Public Health.

REFERENCES

Apter, A., Paasche-Orlow, M. K., Remillard, J. T., Bennett, I. M., Ben-Joseph, E. P., Batista, R., … Rudd, R. E. (2008). Numeracy and communication with patients: They are counting on us. *Journal of General Internal Medicine, 23,* 2117-2124.

Baker, D. W. (2006).The meaning and the measure of health literacy. *Journal of General Internal Medicine, 21*(8), 878-883. doi:10.1111/j.1525-1497.2006.00540.x.

Berkman, N. D., Sheridan, S. L., Donahue, K. E., Halpern, D. J., and Crotty, K. (2011). Low health literacy and health outcomes: An updated systematic review. *Annals of Internal Medicine, 155,* 97-107.

Carroll, L. (1871). *Through the looking glass.* London, England: Macmillan.

Choi, J., and Bakken., S. (2010). Web-based education for low-literate parents in neonatal intensive care unit: Development of a website and heuristic evaluation and usability testing. *International Journal of Medical Informatics, 79,* 565-575.

Davis, T. C., Long, S. W., Jackson, R. H., Mayeaux, E. J., George, R. B., Murphy, P. W., and Crouch, M. A. (1993). Rapid estimate of adult literacy in medicine: A shortened screening instrument. *Family Medicine, 25*, 391-395.

DeWalt, D. A., Berkman, N. D., Sheridan, S., Lohr, K. N., and Pignone, M. P. (2004). Literacy and health outcomes: A systematic review of the literature. *Journal of General Internal Medicine, 19*(12), 1228-1239.

Doak, L. G., Doak, C. C., and Root, J. H. (1996). *Teaching patients with low literacy skills* (2nd ed.). Philadelphia, PA: Lippincott. [Out of print but available with permission at http://www.hsph.harvard.edu/healthliteracy/resources/doak-book/index.html].

Freedman, D. A., Bess, K. D., Tucker, H. A., Boyd, D. L., Tuchman, A. M., and Wallston, K. A. (2009). Public health literacy defined. *American Journal of Preventive Medicine, 36*(5), 446-451.

Friedman, D. B., and Hoffman-Goetz, L. (2006). A systematic review of readability and comprehension instruments used for print and web-based cancer information. *Health Education Behavior, 33*(3), 352-373.

Gazmararian, J. A., Curran, J. W., Parker, R. M., Bernhardt, J. M., and DeBuono, B. A. (2005). Public health literacy in America: An ethical imperative. *American Journal of Preventive Medicine, 28*(3), 317-322.

Groene, O., and Rudd, R. E. (2011). Results of a feasibility study to assess the health literacy environment: Navigation, written and oral communication in ten hospitals in Catalonia, Spain. *Journal of Communication in Healthcare.* 4(4):227-237. 2011.

Grosse, R. N., and Auffrey, C. (1989). Literacy and health status in developing countries. *Annual Review of Public Health, 10,* 281-297.

Harper, W., Cook, S., and Makloul, S. (2007). Teaching medical students about health literacy: 2 Chicago initiatives. *American Journal of Health Behaviour, 31*(S1), S111–114.

Irwin, P. M. (1991). *National Literacy Act of 1991: Major provisions of P.L. 102-73. CRS Report for Congress* (CRS-91-811-EPW). Washington, DC: Congressional Research Service, Library of Congress. Retrieved from ERIC database. (ED341851)

Kirsch, I. S. (2001). *The International Adult Literacy Survey: Understanding what was measured.* Princeton, NJ: Educational Testing Service.

Kirsch, I. S., Jungeblut, A., Jenkins, L., and Kolstad, A. (1993). *Adult literacy in America: The first look at the results of the National Adult Literacy Survey (NALS).* Washington, DC: US Department of Education.

Koch-Weser, S., Rudd, R. E., and DeJong, W. (2010). Quantifying word use to study health literacy in doctor-patient communication. *Journal of Health Communication, 15*, 590-602.

Kutner, M., Greenberg, E., and Baer, J. (2005). *A first look at the literacy of America's adults in the 21ˢᵗ century* (NCES 2006-470). US Department of Education, National Center for Educational Statistics. Washington, DC: US Government Printing Office.

Lee, J. Y., Rozier, R. G., Lee, S. D., Bender, D., and Ruiz, R. E. (2007). Development of a word recognition instrument to test health literacy in dentistry: The REALD-30. *Journal of Public Health Dentistry, 67*(2), 94-98.

Lewin, K. (1943). Defining the "Field at a given time". *Psychological Review. 50*, 292-310.

Martin, L. T., Schonlau, M., Haas, A., Derose, K. P., Rudd, R. E., Loucks, E. B., ... Buka, S. L. (2011). Literacy skills and calculated 10-year risk of coronary heart disease. *Journal of General Internal Medicine, 26*(1), 45-50.

Martin, L. T., Schonlau, M., Haas, A., Derose, K. P., Rosenfeld, L., Buka, S. L., and Rudd, R. E. (2011). Patient activation and advocacy: Which literacy skills matter most? *Journal of Health Communication, 16*(S3), 177-190.

McCray, A. T. (2005). Promoting health literacy. *Journal of American Medical Informatics Association, 12*(2), 152-163.

McCray, A. T. (2006). Conceptualizing the world: Lessons from history. *Journal of Biomedical Informatics, 39*, 267-273.

Mosenthal, P., and Kirsch, I. S. (1998). A new measure for assessing document complexity: The PMOSE/IKIRSCH document readability formula. *Journal of Adolescent and Adult Literacy, 41*, 638-657.

Murray, T. S., Kirsch, I. S., and Jenkins, L. B. (Eds.). (1997). *Adult literacy in OECD countries: Technical report on the First International Adult Literacy Survey* (NCES 98–053). Washington, DC: National Center for Education Statistics.

Nielsen-Bohlman, L., Panzer, A. M., and Kindig, D. A. (Eds.). (2004). *Health literacy: A prescription to end confusion.* Washington, DC: Institute of Medicine of the National Academies and The National Academies Press.

Nutbeam, D. (2000). Health literacy as a public health goal: A challenge for contemporary health education and communication strategies into the 21st century. *Health Promotion International, 15*(3), 259-267.

Nutbeam, D. (2008). The evolving concept of health literacy. *Social Science and Medicine, 67*(12), 2072-2078.

Nutbeam, D., and Wise, M. (1993). Australia: Planning for better health. *Promotion and Education,* 19-24.

Parker, R. M., Baker, D. W., Williams, M. V., and Nurss, J. R. (1995). The test of functional health literacy in adults: A new instrument for measuring patients' literacy skills. *Journal of General Internal Medicine, 10*, 537-541.

Rootman, I., and Gordon-El-Bihbety, D. (2008). *A vision for a health literate Canada: Report of the expert panel on health literacy.* Ottawa, Canada: Canadian Public Health Association.

Rosenfeld, L., Rudd, R. E., Emmons, K., Acevedo-Garcia, D., and Buka S. (2011). Beyond reading alone: Literacy and chronic disease management. *Patient Education and Counseling, 82*(1), 110-116.

Roter, D. L., Erby, L., Larson, S., and Ellington, L. (2007). Assessing oral literacy demand in genetic counseling dialogue: Preliminary test of a conceptual framework. *Social Science and Medicine, 65*, 1442-1457.

Roter, D. L., Erby, L., Larson, S., and Ellington, L. (2009). Oral literacy demand of prenatal genetic counseling dialogue: Predictors of learning. *Patient Education and Counseling, 75,* 392-397.

Rudd, R. E. (2007). Health literacy skills of U.S. adults. *American Journal of Health Behavior, 31*(S1), S8-18.

Rudd, R. E. (2010). Improving Americans' health literacy. *New England Journal of Medicine.* 363, 2283-5.

Rudd, R. E., and Anderson, J. E. (2006). *The health literacy environment of hospitals and health centers: Making your healthcare facility literacy friendly.* Cambridge, MA: National Center for the Study of Adult Learning and Literacy and Health and Adult Literacy and Learning Initiative, Harvard School of Public Health. Available from http://www.ncsall.net/fileadmin/resources/teach/environ.pdf.

Rudd, R. E., Anderson, J. E., Oppenheimer, S., and Nath, C. (2007). Health literacy: An update of public health and medical literature. In J. P. Comings, C. Smith, and B. Garner (Eds.), *Annual review of adult learning and literacy* (pp. 175-204). Mahwah, NJ: Lawrence Erlbaum.

Rudd, R. E., and Keller, D. B. (2009). Health literacy: New developments and research. *Journal of Communication in Healthcare, 2,* 240-257.

Rudd, R. E., Kirsch, I. S., and Yamamoto, K. (2004). *Literacy and health in America* (Policy Information Report). Princeton, NJ: Educational Testing Services.

Rudd, R. E., Moeykens, B. A., and Colton, T. (2000). Health and literacy: A review of the medical and public health literature. In J. P. Comings, C. Smith, and B. Garner (Eds.), *Annual review of adult learning and literacy* (pp. 158-199). San Francisco, CA: Jossey-Bass.

Rudd, R. E., Renzulli, D., Perreira, A., and Daltroy, L. D. (2004). The patients' health experience. In J. G. Schwartzberg et al. (Eds.), *Understanding health literacy: Implications for medicine and public health* (pp. 69-84). Chicago, IL: AMA Press.

Sum, A., Kirsch, I. S., and Taggart, R. (2002). *The twin challenges of mediocrity and inequality: Literacy in the U.S. from an international perspective* (Policy Information Report). Princeton, NJ: Educational Testing Service.

United States Department of Health and Human Services. (2011). *Healthy people 2020*. Washington, DC: Author. Available from http://www.healthypeople.gov.

United States Department of Health and Human Services, Office of Disease Prevention and Health Promotion. (2003). *Communicating health: Priorities and strategies for progress. Action plans to achieve the health communication objectives in Healthy People 2010*. Washington, DC: Author.

United States Department of Health and Human Services, Office of Disease Prevention and Health Promotion. (2010). *National action plan to improve health literacy*. Washington, DC: Author.

United States National Institutes of Health. (2006). *Proceedings of the Surgeon General's workshop on improving health literacy*. Bethesda, MD: Author. Available from http://www.surgeongeneral.gov/topics/health literacy/toc.html.

Weiss, B. D., Mays, M. Z., Martz, W., Castro, K. M., DeWalt, D. A., Pignone, M. P., … Hale, F. A. (2005). Quick assessment of literacy in primary care: The newest vital sign. *Annals of Family Medicine, 3*, 514-522.

World Health Organization. (1998). *Health promotion glossary*. Geneva, Switzerland: Author.

Zarcadoolas, C. (2011). The simplicity complex: Exploring simplified health messages in a complex world. *Health Promotion International, 26*(3), 338-350.

Zarcadoolas, C., Pleasant, A., and Greer, D. S. (2005). Understanding health literacy: An expanded model. *Health Promotion International, 20*(2), 195-203.

In: Health Literacy in Context   ISBN: 978-1-61942-921-5
Eds.: D.Begoray, D.Gillis, G.Rowlands © 2012 Nova Science Publishers, Inc.

Chapter 3

HEALTH LITERACY AND HEALTHY LIFESTYLE CHOICES

Doris E. Gillis and *Nicola J. Gray*

ABSTRACT

Information intended to persuade people to make healthy lifestyle choices abounds from lay and professional, public and private sources within and beyond formal health systems. Positioning the relevant importance of the individual and the broader society in supporting personal health behaviours is central to public health policy and health literacy efforts aimed at improving health outcomes. This chapter examines the multidimensional concepts of health literacy and healthy lifestyle choices within two policy contexts, the United Kingdom and Canada, and from our respective fields of practice, pharmacy and nutrition. By drawing on the literature and examples from our research, we explore ideas about health literacy and the responsibility of individuals for using information to make and act upon an informed choice pertaining to their personal health behaviour.

* Corresponding author: E-mail: dgillis@stfx.ca.

INTRODUCTION

Today's public is expected to assume greater responsibility for their health with much of the health policy discourse centred on enabling individuals to make healthy lifestyle choices. In large part, this expectation comes from the burden placed on health systems by the increasing prevalence of long-term conditions (e.g., obesity and diabetes) and the modifiable risk behaviours associated with them (World Health Organization [WHO], 2008). While it is well recognized that personal behaviours can have a profound impact on one's health, these patterns and one's capacity for changing them depend heavily on circumstances of daily living. This chapter examines health literacy and healthy lifestyle choices within the debate about the relative focus of individual responsibility for healthy lifestyle behaviour versus social responsibility addressing the broader social determinants of health through public policy. We refer to research from our respective fields of practice— pharmacy and nutrition—in examining how various dimensions of health literacy, as conceptualized in the literature, relate to healthy lifestyle choices.

Conceptualizing Healthy Lifestyle

Promoting healthy lifestyles is an important aspect of health promotion, defined as "the process of enabling people to increase control over and to improve their health" (WHO, 1986, p. 1). Although a widely used term, there is no single definition of healthy lifestyle. The elements of choice and of intentional action to prevent disease and enhance health and wellbeing are central to its common usage (Ochieng, 2006). Efforts to promote healthy lifestyle choices tend to imply that individuals are responsible for making and acting upon decisions about their personal health-related behaviours.

WHO (1998) defines lifestyle conducive to health as "a way of living based on identifiable patterns of behaviour which are determined by the interplay between an individual's personal characteristics, social interactions, and socioeconomic and environmental living conditions" (p. 16). The idea that one's freedom of choice may be limited reflects the conflict between one's sense of autonomy and the structural constraints confronted in everyday living. This structure–agency debate is central to health promotion practice and relates to the capacity for choice within the context of one's life chances, that is, the opportunities that exist within one's social situation to shape behaviour (Frohlich and Poland, 2007). "[I]f health is to be improved by engaging individuals to change their lifestyle, action must be directed not only at the individual but also at the social and living conditions which interact to produce and maintain these patterns of behaviour" (WHO, 1998, p. 16). Many authors have argued for greater use of ecological models for health promotion that incorporate attention to healthy lifestyle behaviours within the broader socioeconomic, political, and cultural environment in which people make decisions about health in their daily lives (e.g., Minkler and Wallerstein, 2002; Wharf-Higgins, Begoray, and MacDonald, 2009).

PERSPECTIVES ON THE POLICY CONTEXT SITUATING HEALTHY LIFESTYLE CHOICES AND HEALTH LITERACY

The understanding and application of concepts such as healthy lifestyle choices and health literacy depend largely upon the health policy context and extent to which health is viewed as a personal or societal responsibility. To exemplify this, we present perspectives on health literacy as it relates to healthy lifestyle choices within two policy contexts, that of the United Kingdom (UK) and of Canada.

United Kingdom Context

In the UK, the responsibility of members of the public to make healthy lifestyle choices in order to make best use of formal health services was emphasized by the fully engaged scenario described in the report *Securing Good Health for the Whole Population* (Wanless, 2004) and the National Health Service (NHS) Constitution (Department of Health, England [DHE], 2009). Our discussion of health literacy is considered within the UK definition of public health as "the science and art of preventing disease, prolonging life and promoting health through the organised efforts and informed choices of society, organisations, public and private, communities and individuals" (Wanless, 2004, p. 3). More recently, the coalition administration elected in 2010 has championed "The Responsibility Deal," which involves "positively promoting 'healthier' behaviours and lifestyles among individuals; adapting the environment to make healthy choices easier; and strengthening self-esteem, confidence, and personal responsibility" (DHE, 2011, p. 3). There is a strong emphasis, consistent with conservative ideology, on involving private companies in public endeavours. It is noteworthy that the Marmot Review (Marmot, 2010) commented upon the limited effectiveness of trying to change individual behaviours without acting upon the wider social context with an emphasis on public policy.

Various definitions of health literacy have appeared in national policy documents in the last decade. Britain's National Consumer Council (NCC) adopted the 1991 USA Joint Committee on National Health Education Standards definition of health literacy as "the capacity of an individual to obtain, interpret, and understand basic health information and services and the competence to use such information and services in ways which are health-enhancing" (Sihota and Lennard, 2004, p. 5). Although the NCC's report firmly anchors health literacy within the health care context, it points to "a need to develop a broader-based investigation that goes beyond medically determined studies to include sociological research. This is vital in order to look specifically at differences between groups in decision-making capacity and preferences" (Sihota and Lennard, 2004, p. 7).

Health literacy concepts are implicit, rather than explicit, in many UK policy documents relating to healthy lifestyle choices, such as the Marmot Review (2010). Similarly, the Wanless Review (2004) of the long-term future for health services showcased a fully engaged scenario, where people would make appropriate and prudent use of health services because they took responsibility for their and their family's health by adopting healthy lifestyle behaviours. The rights and responsibilities of individuals were juxtaposed in the NHS Constitution (DHE, 2009). Age Concern's (now Age UK; 2006) *As Fit As Butchers' Dogs?* report cited poor health literacy as a contributing factor in practical challenges to compliance with healthy behaviours but not in challenges relating to health beliefs, which perhaps reflects a narrow view of the concept.

The Labour Government's *Choosing Health through Pharmacy* (DHE, 2005) highlighted health literacy as a tool to reduce health inequalities. The document had specific recommendations for improving health literacy and designating pharmacists as health-literate employers through the training of pharmacy staff. DHE has had quite sophisticated health literacy policy in a public health context, not least because Don Nutbeam was the Head of Public Health from 2000–03. Since 2010, the coalition government has introduced subtle changes in public health policy; and the structure of public health practice is undergoing reorganisation (DHE, 2010). Industry is partnering with government to develop public health policy, and the concept of nudging, rather than nannying, summarises the current administration's preference and ideology that the public take responsibility for their own health. This approach refers to "the claim that it is legitimate for choice architects to try to influence people's behaviour in order to make their lives longer, healthier, and better" (Thaler and Sunstein, 2008, p. 5).

The academic and practitioner discourse on health literacy is very limited. Some primary care organisations (local health management systems) are using the term in documents but with a very narrow focus on readable leaflets and other functional activities. The main vehicle for improving health literacy has been a family-based, adult learning program called "Skilled for Health." This program involved a partnership between the Department of Health; the Department for Business, Innovation, and Skills; and the learning and health charity ContinYou (see Chapter 5 for more on Skilled for Health). Many of the learning units incorporated healthy lifestyle information, such as healthy eating, alcohol intake, and exercising. The final evaluation (Tavistock Institute and Shared Intelligence, 2009) of the project reported positive primary health outcomes for participants in terms of taking exercise and healthy eating; in addition, it reported secondary outcomes of participants cascading their learned information back into their families and communities.

Canadian Context

In Canada, there has been considerable debate on the relative emphasis on individual lifestyle in contrast to social environmental approaches to health promotion (Frohlich and Poland, 2007). Whereas an ecological model based upon social determinants of health underpins the Public Health Agency of Canada's Population Health Approach, an individualized lifestyle approach appears to prevail in public health practice. Raphael (2007, 2008), for instance, has argued that Canadian public health practitioners place too much emphasis on modifying lifestyle practices and not enough on effecting public policy change to improve social determinants of health. Raphael has challenged policy makers and practitioners to refocus their orientation from promoting healthy lifestyle behaviours toward addressing the root causes of health disparities. As noted by Alvaro et al. (2010), "government policies are, for the most part, 'stuck' at promoting individual lifestyle change" (p. 91).

The appearance of health literacy as an issue of interest in Canada stemmed in large part from recognition of literacy as a key determinant of health having both direct and indirect impacts on health outcomes (Ronson and Rootman, 2009). In contrast to the USA where attention to health literacy tended to be within the context of interactions between medical providers and their patients in clinical care settings, there has been relatively little interest in health literacy among Canadian medical practitioners (Rootman, 2006). Canadian leaders in health literacy have leaned toward a public health approach firmly rooted in health promotion thinking and a concern about both literacy and health literacy as social determinants of health (Rootman, Frankish, and Kaszap, 2007).

This broader view of health literacy can largely be attributed to the collaboration and dialogue of leaders from the fields of health and adult education/literacy (Rootman and Ronson, 2005). Notably, this perspective on health literacy has emerged despite the Canadian policy context for literacy. Researchers in literacy have pointed out that a functional view of literacy has tended to dominate policy and practice. In a review of the state of the field of adult literacy, prepared for the Canadian Council on Learning's Health and Learning Knowledge Centre, Quigley, Folinsbee, and Kraglund-Gauthier (2006) claimed that Canadian literacy organizations tended to focus primarily on basic adult literacy skills to the exclusion of other dimensions of literacy. According to Shohet (2004), emphasis on the assessment of population literacy and health literacy reinforced the idea of functional literacy implicit in operational definitions of literacy and health literacy underlying these measures. As Shohet (2004) noted, "Many policy initiatives are caught between the political demand for quantifiable, measurable outcomes, and the recognition that literacy is a complex, multifaceted issue that cuts across many domains" (p. 66).

In 2008, the Expert Panel on Health Literacy, convened by the Canadian Public Health Association and funded by the Canadian Council on Learning, released its report entitled *A Vision for a Health Literate Canada* (Rootman and Gordon-El-Bihbety, 2008). Based on a 2-year examination of data and wide consultation, the Panel concluded that "[L]ow health literacy is a serious and costly problem that will likely grow as the population ages and the incidence of chronic disease increases." (Rootman and Gordon-El-Bihbety, 2008, p. 43). The Panel defined health literacy as, "the ability to access, understand, evaluate and communicate information as a way to promote, maintain and improve health in a variety of settings across the life-course" (p. 11). While this definition spoke to the essential role of health literacy in enabling individuals to take control of and manage their health, the report emphasized that both individuals and society have a role to play in promoting health literacy. This view of health literacy extends beyond the ability and skills of individuals to include the interaction of people and systems, including providers of information within these systems. The report pointed to a number of individual and systemic barriers to health literacy. Increasingly, health literacy is seen as an important contributor to the health of Canadians with the extent and distribution of health literacy linked to health disparities.

MULTIPLE DIMENSIONS OF HEALTH LITERACY IN THE LITERATURE

Given the different paradigms from which health policies and practices are derived, it is not surprising that competing perspectives on health literacy are described in the literature (see Chapter 2). These various understandings are important in applying the multidimensional concept of health literacy to the promotion of healthy lifestyle choices.

Early conceptualization of health literacy tended to refer to the ability of individuals to access, understand, and use information within predominantly clinical health care settings, often with the goal of increasing compliance with medical instructions (Peerson and Saunders, 2009). More recently, it has expanded to encompass the wide range of settings in which people make decisions about their health—both within and outside health care systems. Because choices about healthy living are made primarily outside health care settings, it is especially important to recognize the importance of varied settings and contexts in relating health literacy to healthy lifestyle choices (Kickbusch, Maag, and Saan, 2005).

An important turning point in conceptualizing health literacy was acknowledgement that individual decision making is heavily influenced by the social systems and structures that determine health, within both individual and broader community and societal contexts (Nielsen-Bohlman, Panzer, and Kindig, 2004). As emphasized in a landmark report by the US Institute of Medicine's Committee on Health Literacy, "health literacy is a shared function of social and individual factors" (Nielsen-Bohlman et al., 2004, p. 4). Increasingly, health literacy is seen not primarily as a deficit in skills of potential users of health information but rather as the unique set of skills and capacity of both users and providers of information. Nutbeam (2008) described health literacy as an asset—a concept closely aligned with the WHO definition of health literacy:

> Health literacy represents the cognitive and social skills which determine
> the motivation and ability of individuals to gain access to, understand, and
> use information in ways which promote and maintain good health .... [By]
> improving people's access to health information and their capacity to use it
> effectively, health literacy is seen as critical to personal empowerment.
> (WHO, 1998, p. 10)

Whereas personal empowerment and control over one's health are admirable goals, placing sole responsibility on individuals for making informed choices consistent with healthy lifestyles can be viewed as often unattainable for those living in circumstances that constrain them from taking action on advice provided. "Culture, income, family structure, age, physical ability, home and work environment will make certain ways and conditions of living more attractive, feasible and appropriate" (WHO, 1998, p. 16).

Nutbeam (1999) proposed a health literacy typology comprised of three levels that "progressively allow for greater autonomy and personal empowerment" (p. 50). In combination, these three types of health literacy reinforce the view that lifestyle behaviours are determined by personal traits of individuals, their interaction with others, and the socioeconomic and environmental circumstances of daily living. These levels are basic/functional, communicative/interactive, and critical literacy.

Basic/functional health literacy is characterized as "sufficient basic skills in reading and writing to be able to function effectively in everyday situations" (Nutbeam, 2000, p. 263). Functional health literacy tends to focus on one's command over the written word and, more commonly, the lack of literacy skills. In health practice, this focus has tended to place priority on providing easy-to-understand health information to individuals, often with the goal of compliance through personal behavioural changes.

Communicative/interactive health literacy refers to "more advanced cognitive and literacy skills which, together with social skills, can be used to actively participate in everyday activities, to extract information and derive meaning from different forms of communication, and to apply new information to changing circumstances" (Nutbeam, 2000, pp. 263–264). An interactive health literacy approach aims to move individuals beyond their understanding of information to enhancing their capacity to act on information provided, in particular through improved motivation and self-confidence. Beyond benefits to the individual, social benefits can be derived through one's improved capacity to interact with social groups and to influence social norms.

The development of personal and social skills is central to influencing adoption of healthy lifestyle practices at the individual and population level.

Critical health literacy encompasses "advanced cognitive skills which, together with social skills, can be applied to critically analyse information, and to use this information to exert greater control over life events and situations" (Nutbeam, 2000, p. 264). Two traditions of criticality are embedded in his notion of critical health literacy—one of critical appraisal of information and one of emancipation. The first is relevant to making healthy lifestyle choices, especially given the wide array of health messages from multiple sources and channels directed to today's public. The second notion of critical health literacy moves beyond the communication of information to the development of skills needed to effect social change. By improving individual and community capacity to understand and address the social and economic determinants of health, Nutbeam (2000) posits that critical health literacy can benefit the larger population, for example, by making it easier to adopt healthier lifestyle practices. Chinn (2011) recently explored some of the complexities of critical health literacy and its usefulness as a "social asset which helps individuals towards a critical engagement with health information" (p. 60).

Nutbeam (2000) noted that, in practice, efforts consistent with enhancing health literacy are typically based on a mixture of these three types of literacy, with critical health literacy the least commonly applied. This critical dimension of health literacy has particular relevance to public health practice and policy given the growing concern for addressing health inequalities and eliminating social inequities. Increasingly, importance is placed on broadening the focus of health literacy to take into account the barriers to acting on information posed by the socioeconomic context in which people live. According to the report from the WHO Commission on Social Determinants of Health (2008), understandings of health literacy should be expanded to include the ability to access, understand, evaluate, and communicate information on the social determinants of health. Freedman, Bess, Tucker, Boyd, Tuchman, and Wallston (2009) defined public health literacy as more than an individual-level construct, rather one that takes into account "the complex social, ecologic, and systemic forces affecting health and well-being" (p. 46); they emphasized the importance of health literacy in making public health decisions that benefit the community as a whole.

Many Roles, Many Literacies

Kickbusch (2009) stated that health literacy is one of the most critical capabilities in modern society as it "can empower and enable people to make sound health decisions in the context of everyday life – at home, in the community, at the workplace, in the health care system, in the marketplace, and – above all – in the political arena" (p. 132). That individuals are expected to draw on their health literacy ability in different settings and contexts when engaging with diverse forms and sources of information relevant to their health suggests multiple dimensions of health literacy. Zarcadoolas, Pleasant, and Greer (2006) described health literacy as "the wide range of skills and competencies that people develop over their lifetimes to seek out, comprehend, evaluate, and use health information and concepts to make informed choices, reduce health risks, and increase quality of life" (p. 76); their expanded model for health literacy is comprised of four literacy domains: fundamental, scientific, cultural, and civic. This idea of multiple literacies is also reflected in the concept of eHealth literacy coined by Norman and Skinner (2006), as "the ability to seek, find, understand, and appraise health information from electronic sources and apply the knowledge gained to addressing or solving a health problem" (p. 2). In their eHealth literacy model, they integrated six different types of literacy: literacy, health literacy, information literacy, scientific literacy, media literacy, and computer literacy.

In summary, the multiple dimensions of health literacy suggested by Nutbeam (2000), Zarcadoolas et al. (2006), and Skinner and Norman (2006) highlight important aspects of a broadly constructed notion of health literacy as it pertains to healthy lifestyle choices.

- Health literacy refers to the ability of both individuals and the varied systems in which they interact with information relevant to healthy living.
- There are many and varied contexts and settings in which people are expected to access, understand, communicate, and evaluate information in order to make informed choices.
- Engaging with health information in contemporary society to make healthy lifestyle choices requires a range of literacy and health literacy skills.
- The context of everyday life weighs heavily on people's capacity to use information, not only to make an informed choice but to take action that is consistent with healthy living.

- Both individual and social benefits to building health literacy capacity related to supporting healthy lifestyle choices should be considered.

Peerson and Saunders (2009), among others, have suggested that more attention be given to the broader conceptualization and operationalization of health literacy and its multiple dimensions.

LESSONS FROM THE FIELD

A small number of more recent studies on health literacy interventions address healthy lifestyle practices among diverse population groups at various life stages and within varying contexts and settings (e.g., von Wagner, Knight, Steptoe, and Wardle, 2007; Lee, Tsai, Tsai, and Kuo, 2011). In their latest systematic review of the literature, Berkman et al. (2011) found mixed results in the relationship between health literacy and healthy lifestyle practices. The eight studies meeting their inclusion criteria reported using various measures of healthy lifestyle for physical activity, eating habits, and seatbelt use. They identified a lack of measurement tools that take into account the diversity in settings and contexts of health literacy interventions as a major challenge in evaluating such interventions.

Abel (2008) argued that different measures of health literacy are needed for various types of interventions and that consideration must be given to whether health literacy interventions are intended to contribute to health through medical services or through lifestyle modification. According to Nutbeam (2009), measures need to be developed that take into account health content and contexts as well as different ages and stages across the life course. The long-established tools REALM (Davis et al., 1993) and s-TOFHLA (Baker, Williams, Parker, Gazmararian, and Nurss, 1999) reflect a health service emphasis, but newer tools like the Newest Vital Sign (Weiss et al., 2005) draw upon skills reflecting everyday health (and, in that case, nutrition) decisions. As noted by Rootman (2009), none of the existing tools to measure general literacy or health literacy fully measure all dimensions of definitions noted in the literature. Given the early stage in development of health literacy measurement tools, particularly those that operationalise a broad, multifaceted understanding of health literacy, it is not surprising that few reports of interventions demonstrate rigorous methods of evaluation (King, 2007).

The pharmacy and nutrition/dietetic sectors of health practice, not hitherto predominant in reports of health literacy research, have much to offer in understanding the contribution of health literacy to the goal of promoting healthy lifestyle choices. Through these two professional perspectives, we uncover some of the tensions underpinning ideas about health literacy and healthy lifestyle choices.

Case Study 1: Young People's Use of Online Health Information

Young people are the parents and caregivers of the near future; they are crucial to the future health of our society and to make appropriate use of health services. They form a key user group of the Internet—they use it to make sense of most things in their world. Information about any subject is readily available from a range of sources. In the YouthNet's Life Support survey (Hulme, 2009), young people aged 16–24 cited parents and the Internet as their preferred health information sources. Commentators and educators assume that most young people are skilled Internet users, but we would argue that there is another insidious digital divide relating to the experience users have online (Gray, Klein, Cantrill, and Noyce, 2002). One study has shown people rate their Internet search experience highly, despite a poor success rate (Zeng et al., 2004).

In 2001–02, we explored Internet use for health and medicines information through focus groups with 160 young people aged 11–18 years in the UK and the US (Gray, Klein, Noyce, Sesselberg, and Cantrill, 2005a, 2005b). We did not initially undertake the research to explore health literacy, but the challenges that participants reported when finding health information online emerged as potential health literacy issues. Each group was asked to find some information about a health-related issue of their choice. One member of the group sat at an Internet-linked computer and acted as the navigator; the other group members directed the navigator's actions.

Our findings reflected the dimensions of Nutbeam's tripartite model of health literacy (2000). Functional health literacy challenges included difficulty spelling search terms and constructing coherent search queries. One group of young men wanted to search for information about gonorrhoea, but none knew how to spell the word. A plaintive cry from one group member to *Search for something you can spell* signalled the end of that particular quest. Another group was interested in information about good sleep habits for children and young people; they had difficulty, however, in constructing a pithy search term that would clearly articulate their particular interest. This led to them choosing but quickly rejecting sites from the results and going back to change the search term to make their results more relevant.

Critical health literacy challenges included knowing which sources to trust and dealing with information overload. Comments from participants about buying medicines online, for example, included perceptions that it was safer to buy from sites that had an offline presence, such as online extensions of bricks-and-mortar pharmacy chains (Gray et al., 2002). Young people reported cross-checking of information, both across different sites and against other sources of information such as parents, in order to judge its credibility. The analysis of website addresses, such as the use of the ending *.edu*, was reported as another strategy for determining trustworthiness.

Interactive health literacy challenges reflected a difficulty in acting upon information, for example, finding local sources of help and knowing what to do next. Sometimes no action was the desired endpoint; one young man reported using the Internet to find out more about creatine as a sport supplement and decided not to use it because of the information that he found. This was an example of an increase in self-confidence that empowered a health decision. Several young people reported using the Internet for diet and fitness information and the adoption of healthy behaviours; they liked the option to personalise this information through filling in surveys. Again, this required little interaction with offline health providers to put information into action. The crunch came when someone else's help was needed to make the action count. This might be the case for alcohol harm reduction or smoking cessation. Young people needed to know whom to contact in their locality.

The exploration of our findings in terms of multiple literacies and e-health literacy was not explored at the time of original work (which pre-dates them), but it is possible now to re-examine our results to see reflections of these different aspects of health literacy. The concept of civic literacy within the Zarcadoolas et al. (2006) model can be applied to the recognised restrictions on use of the Internet for health information in public places and the content filters on public computers that can block health content about sexual health issues. Cultural literacy can be reflected in young people knowing the meaning of site addresses (e.g., *co.uk* being associated with commercial websites). Scientific literacy underpins their understanding of medical jargon on health sites.

The application of health literacy theory to the use of the Internet fits with the notion of health literacy as an asset (Nutbeam, 2008). Proficiency in these skills would help young people to determine information credibility and to develop strategies to prevent information overload.

Case Study 2: Health Literacy and the Promotion of Breastfeeding

Canadian women are considered important gatekeepers for health information and influential in promoting health in their families (Ostry, 2006). Breastfeeding has been a longstanding public health priority (Nathoo and Ostry, 2009) with Canadian breastfeeding efforts directed to enabling women to make an informed choice (Knack, 2006). This focus is in keeping with a key objective of the Global Strategy for Infant and Young Child Feeding "to create an environment that will enable mothers, families and other caregivers in all circumstances to make—and implement—informed choices about the optimal feeding practices for infants and young children" (WHO, 2003, p. 7).

In 2005–06, a case study examined the extent to which breastfeeding promotion practices reflected dimensions of health literacy. It was conducted in northeastern Nova Scotia, a health district where breastfeeding initiation and duration rates as well as reported levels of health literacy are lower than national and provincial averages. The study was undertaken within the context of two district-wide policies. One supported national and provincial level policy to position breastfeeding as the cultural norm; the other was developed in response to local research findings (Gillis, Quigley, and MacIsaac, 2005; Gillis and Sears, 2011) and positioned health literacy as an important determinant of health.

Thirty lay and professional practitioners were interviewed about their breastfeeding promotion practices. Practices were observed in one hospital and two community health sites. To solicit input on preliminary findings, group interviews were held with two groups of mothers and two groups of practitioners who had been individually interviewed. Data were analyzed for themes reflecting dimensions of health literacy in the current literature (Nutbeam, 2000; Zarcadoolas et al., 2006); four domains emerged from the analyses.

Functional Health Literacy

A large amount of print-based information on breastfeeding was found to be directed to mothers. At the time, the provincial government was revising their resources to address the literacy needs of parents. Although practitioners described situations that required their clients to apply functional literacy skills, few practitioners appeared aware of their clients' functional health literacy capacity. As one hospital maternity nurse said, *We just assume that everybody can read that pamphlet that we hand them—which knowing the literacy levels of the community, we know not to be true* (P1, 112). Many comments reflected the stigma attached to low literacy plus practitioners' discomfort and reluctance to address literacy concerns with their clients.

Interactive Health Literacy

Practitioners considered their personal interactions with women key to their role in promoting and supporting breastfeeding. Most stressed the importance of providing information about breastfeeding when meeting with women. As noted by one public health nutritionist, *I think we go with this, 'well, let's just go and provide them with all of the information' instead of maybe starting with what do they need to know and having a conversation* (P2, 27). Many practitioners referred to their role in helping mothers make an informed choice during these interactions. Commonly, an informed choice implied breastfeeding. This assumption was most explicitly stated during a practitioners' group interview: *Because that is what we want them to do, make an informed choice ... the informed choice that they are going to make is breastfeeding* (FG 2). The pressure placed on mothers to at least give breastfeeding a try reflected the importance placed on encouraging mothers to act on the informed choice—to breastfeed. The guilt expressed by mothers who did not maintain breastfeeding according to the advice of their practitioners was a striking and recurring theme.

Critical Health Literacy

Many practitioners talked about the inconsistent information mothers received from various sources. There was little mention, however, of practices aimed at enabling women to assess the credibility of sources, appraise conflicting information, or assess the pros and cons of feeding options through information provided. A primary health care nurse said, *It is definitely biased towards breastfeeding, the information you receive. It is not an equal choice people* [practitioners] *are giving people. We don't talk about the benefits of formula; we only talk of the benefits of breast milk* (P6, 283). Despite considerable discussion of the socioeconomic and cultural constraints to breastfeeding in this rural district, little reference was made to actions to reduce structural barriers preventing women from acting on their informed choice to breastfeed. This finding is consistent with reports in the literature that practices reflecting critical health literacy are least likely to be seen (Nutbeam, 2000).

Multiple Health Literacies

Practitioners appeared to give little attention to helping mothers develop or apply scientific literacy, such as by comparing the health benefits and risks of breastfeeding and bottle feeding. Many did, however, identify the widespread use of scientific terms associated with lactation as problematic. For example, one family physician said, *I am sure a lot of them would not know what colostrum was, for instance, so I mean, you could explain* (P19, 126). Notably, some practitioners suggested that their clients did not want technical information. Although practitioners frequently mentioned taboos to breastfeeding in public places (and in private homes), their comments did not reflect the application of cultural literacy in breaking through cultural barriers. Similarly, few examples of practices reflected civic literacy. Of note, however, was one practitioner's description of how she supported a small group of parents advocating for breastfeeding-friendly space after a breastfeeding mother and her baby were asked to leave a local restaurant. Whereas practitioners appeared to draw upon their multiple literacies as they talked about their challenges promoting breastfeeding (e.g., scientific literacy in explaining lactation), there was little mention of practices reflecting efforts to enhance mothers' skills. This finding is not surprising given the emphasis practitioners placed on transmitting information to encourage women to breastfeed with less consideration for how women might develop the capacity to act upon this information within the context and constraints of their lives.

Looking through the multifaceted lens of health literacy at breastfeeding, an example of a healthy lifestyle choice, surfaced the tension between individual and societal responsibility implicit in the notion of informed choice. Findings suggested a redirection in practice is needed with less focus on transmitting information persuading women to breastfeed and more attention to addressing the personal, social, and economic constraints that prevent women from acting on information provided. A capacity-building approach consistent with interactive and critical health literacy and multiple literacies may be more effective than the deficit approach implicit in functional health literacy.

CONCLUSION

According to Woolf et al. (2005), one of "the great ironies of the modern health care system is how poorly it delivers knowledge at a time when society enjoys unprecedented access to information" (p. 293). Although many individuals want to be informed about their options and participate in decision making, the system and providers within it may not be equipped to support individuals adequately so as to help them select their best option. Incorporating understandings of health literacy into practice may be of use to providers as they work with individuals to promote healthy lifestyle choices through ways that focus not only on information provision but also on development of health literacy skills.

Traditional health service thinking that exists about health literacy is geared to accommodating poor health literacy (often aimed at those with low literacy), reflecting the *deficit* approach, by simplifying information and communicating it in different ways. There is a fundamental difference in the practice approach needed to promote better health literacy, consistent with the *asset* approach; providers need to take every opportunity to support the development of transferable skills that people can use in different situations. Providing health information is clearly not enough.

The challenge for the health system, as it relates to promoting and supporting healthy lifestyle choices, is that many of the decisions are influenced and taken well beyond the reach and influence of providers. That is one reason why the asset approach is so important. For example, the decision whether or not to breastfeed is arguably formed well before the first interaction with health services during pregnancy; powerful forces of longstanding cultural norms and civic practices may not be swayed by well-meaning advice and leaflets from professionals. The promotion of healthy lifestyle choices across the life course requires a concerted public health effort—one that recognizes the connection between lifestyle practices and the broader social determinants of health. The population groups highlighted in this chapter—young people and new mothers—are important groups to influence in order to move toward a fully engaged scenario promoted by policy makers.

An understanding of the multiple dimensions of health literacy has something to offer to practitioners in their struggle to promote healthy lifestyle choices. If there is any doubt in the minds of clients about the true element of *choice* in communication with providers, the concepts of interactive and critical health literacy are suppressed; as well, the basis for a future, trusting relationship within which an honest discussion can take place about the relative risks and benefits of different lifestyle behaviours is compromised. Providers will be marginalised from those they most want to influence in addressing healthy lifestyle practices and, ultimately, redressing health disparities.

Defining health literacy broadly and identifying its multiple facets not only emphasizes the importance of context but also suggests that we rethink our ways of practice. New ways of thinking about the promotion of healthy lifestyle behaviours—and assumptions about acting on an informed choice— become an imperative when working with those living in communities where socioeconomic and cultural conditions of everyday living present barriers to adopting healthy behaviours. The context of one's life determines one's capacity to act on an informed choice and to adopt a healthy lifestyle. As noted by Director-General Dr. Margaret Chan (2008) at the launch of the final report of the WHO Commission on Social Determinants of Health, "Lifestyles are important determinants of health. But ... it is factors in the social environment that determine access to health services and influence lifestyle choices in the first place." (para. 6–7).

There is a need for research directed to examining health literacy as it relates to the complexities of healthy lifestyle choice and social determinants of health. As noted in the UK's Wanless Review and Canada's Expert Panel on Health Literacy report, rigorous implementation and evaluation of interventions are lacking. While much remains to be learned about its operationalisation, the multifaceted concept of health literacy holds much promise for enabling practitioners and policy makers to rethink the promotion of healthy lifestyle choices with its focus on individual responsibility for self-care and the implicit assumption that individuals will act on an informed choice.

Questions for Further Reflection

We ask readers to consider the following questions as they reflect on their experiences both as providers and users of health information:

1) What do you see as the challenges and opportunities to using a health literacy *lens* in explaining and informing healthy lifestyle issues and interventions?

2) What are the implications for future practice and policy development related to the idea of individual responsibility and promoting healthy lifestyle choices?

3) Is it actually possible to make healthy choices when living in a community with overwhelming social and economic constraints to healthy living? In what ways might healthy choices in these conditions be achieved?

4) Are efforts to enhance health literacy of benefit to individuals or are they further contributing to marginalization and health inequalities? How might this issue be addressed?

REFERENCES

Abel, T. (2008). Measuring health literacy: Moving towards a health-promotion perspective. *International Journal of Public Health, 53*(4), 169-170.

Age Concern England. (2006). *As fit as butchers' dogs?—A report on healthy lifestyle choice and older people.* London, England: Age Concern Reports. Available from http://www.ageuk.org.uk/documents/en-gb/for-professionals/health-and-wellbeing/494_0206_as_fit_as_butchers%E2%80%99_dogs_a_report_on_healthy_lifestyle_choice_and_older_people_2006_pro.pdf?dtrk=true.

Alvaro, C., Jackson, L. A., Kirk, S., McHugh, T. L., Hughes, J., Chircop, A., and Lyons, R. F. (2010). Moving Canadian government policies beyond a focus on individual lifestyle: Some insights from complexity and critical theories. *Health Promotional International, 26*(1), 91-99.

Baker, D. W., Williams, M. V., Parker, R. M., Gazmararian, J. A., and Nurss, J. (1999). Development of a short test to measure functional health literacy. *Patient Education and Counselling, 38*, 33-42.

Berkman, N. D., Sheridan, S. L., Donahue, K. E., Halpern, D. J., Viera, A., Crotty, K.,...Viswanathan, M. (2011, March). *Health literacy interventions and outcomes: An updated systematic review* (Evidence Report /Technology Assessment No. 199; AHRQ Publication Number 11-E006). Rockville, MD: Agency for Healthcare Research and Quality.

Chan, M. (2008). *Comments at the launch of the final report of the World Health Organization Commission Social Determinants of Health.* Retrieved from http://www.who.int/dg/speeches/2008/20080828/en/index.html.

Chinn, D. (2011). Critical health literacy: A review and critical analysis. *Social Science and Medicine, 73*, 60-67.

Commission on Social Determinants of Health. (2008). *Closing the gap in a generation: Health equity through action on the social determinants of health.* Geneva, Switzerland: World Health Organization Commission.

Davis, T. C., Long, S. W., Jackson, R. H., Mayeaux, E. J., George, R. B., Murphy, P. W., and Crouch, M. A. (1993). Rapid estimate of adult literacy in medicine: A shortened screening instrument. *Family Medicine, 25*, 391-395.

Department of Health, England. (2005). *Choosing health through pharmacy: A programme for pharmaceutical public health 2005–2015.* London, England: Author. Available from http://www.dh.gov.uk/prod_consum_dh/groups/dh_digitalassets/@dh/@en/documents/digitalasset/dh_4107496.pdf.

Department of Health, England. (2009). *The NHS constitution for England.* London, England: Author. Available from http://www.dh.gov.uk/en/Publicationsandstatistics/Publications/PublicationsPolicyAndGuidance/DH_093419.

Department of Health, England. (2010). *Healthy lives, healthy people: Our strategy for public health in England* [White paper]. London, England: Author. Available from http://www.dh.gov.uk/en/Publicationsandstatistics/Publications/PublicationsPolicyAndGuidance/DH_121941.

Department of Health, England. (2011). *The public health responsibility deal.* London, England: Author. Available from http://www.dh.gov.uk/prod_consum_dh/groups/dh_digitalassets/documents/digitalasset/dh_125237.pdf.

Freedman, D. A., Bess, K. D., Tucker, H. A., Boyd, D. L., Tuchman, A. M., and Wallston, K. A. (2009). Public health literacy defined. *American Journal of Preventive Medicine, 36*(5), 446-451.

Frohlich, K., and Poland, B. (2007). Points of intervention in health promotion practice. In M. O'Neill, A. Pederson, S. Dupere, and I. Rootman (Eds.), *Health promotion in Canada: Critical perspectives* (2nd ed., pp. 46-60). Toronto, Ontario: Canadian Scholar's Press.

Gillis, D. E., Quigley, B. A., and MacIsaac, A. (2005). "If you were me, how could you make it better?": Responding to the challenge of literacy and health. *Literacies, 5*, 28-31.

Gillis, D. E., and Sears, S. A. (2011). Health literacy in rural communities: Challenges and champions. In J. C. Kulig and A. M. Williams (Eds.), *Health in rural Canada* (pp. 209-224). Vancouver, Canada: UBC Press.

Gray, N. J., Klein, J. D., Cantrill, J. A., and Noyce, P. R. (2002). Adolescent girls' use of the Internet for health information: Issues beyond access. *Journal of Medical Systems, 26*, 545-553.

Gray, N. J., Klein, J. D., Noyce, P. R., Sesselberg, T. S., and Cantrill, J. A. (2005a). Health information-seeking behaviour in adolescence: The place of the Internet. *Social Science and Medicine, 60*(7), 1467-1478.

Gray, N. J., Klein, J. D., Noyce, P. R., Sesselberg, T. S., and Cantrill, J. A. (2005b). The Internet: A window on adolescent health literacy. *Journal of Adolescent Health, 37*, 243.e1-243.e7.

Hulme, M. (2009). *Life support: Young people's needs in a digital age.* London, England: YouthNet UK. Available from http://www.youthnet. org/wp-content/uploads/2011/05/Life-Support-Report.pdf.

Kickbusch, I. S. (2009). Health literacy: Engaging in a political debate. *International Journal of Public Health, 54*(3), 131-132.

Kickbusch, I. S., Maag, D., and Saan, H. (2005, October). *Enabling healthy choices in modern health societies.* Paper presented at the European Health Forum on Partnerships for Health, Badgastein, Austria. Retrieved from http://www.ilonakickbusch.com/health-literacy.

King, J. (2007). *Environmental scan of interventions to improve health literacy: Final report.* Antigonish, Canada: National Collaborating Centre for Determinants of Health. Retrieved from http://www.nccdh.ca/ supportfiles/NCCDH_EnvScanLiteracy_Sep909.pdf.

Knaak, S. (2006). The problem with breastfeeding discourse. *Canadian Journal of Public Health, 97*(5), 412-414.

Lee, S-Y. D., Tsai, T-I., Tsai, Y-W., and Kuo, K. N. (2011). Health literacy and women's health-related behaviours in Taiwan. *Health Education and Behavior.* Advance online publication. doi:10.1177/1090198111413126.

Marmot, M. (2010). *Fair society, healthy lives: Strategic review of health inequalities in England post-2010.* London, England: The Marmot Review Team. Retrieved from www.marmotreview.org.

Minkler, M., and Wallerstein, N. B. (2002). Improving health through community organization and community building. In K. Glanz, B. K. Rimer, and F. M. Lewis (Eds.), *Health behavior and health education: Theory, practice and research* (pp. 279-311). San Francisco, CA: Wiley.

Nathoo, T., and Ostry, A. (2009). *The one best way? Breastfeeding history, politics, and policy in Canada.* Waterloo, Canada: Wilfrid Laurier University Press.

Nielsen-Bohlman, L., Panzer, A. M., and Kindig, D. A. (Eds.). (2004). *Health literacy: A prescription to end confusion.* Washington, DC: Institute of Medicine of the National Academies and The National Academies Press.

Norman, C. D., and Skinner, H. A. (2006). eHealth literacy: Essential skills for consumer health in a networked world. *Journal of Medical Internet Research, 8*(2), e9. doi:10.2196/jmir.8.2.e9.

Nutbeam, D. (1999). Literacies across the lifespan: Health literacy. *Literacy and Numeracy Studies, 9*(2), 47-56.

Nutbeam, D. (2000). Health literacy as a public health goal: A challenge for contemporary health education and communication strategies into the 21st century. *Health Promotion International, 15*(3), 259-267.

Nutbeam, D. (2008).The evolving concept of health literacy. *Social Science and Medicine, 67*(12), 2072-2078.

Nutbeam, D. (2009). Defining and measuring health literacy: What can we learn from literacy studies? *International Journal of Public Health, 54*, 303-305.

Ochieng, B. (2006). Factors affecting choice of a healthy lifestyle: Implications for nurses. *British Journal Community Nursing, 11*(2), 78-81.

Ostry, A. S. (2006). *Nutrition policy in Canada, 1870-1939.* Vancouver, Canada: UBC Press.

Peerson, A., and Saunders, M. (2009). Health literacy revisited: What do we mean and why does it matter? *Health Promotion International, 24*, 285-296.

Quigley, B. A., Folinsbee, S., and Kraglund-Gauthier, W. L. (2006). *State of the field report on adult literacy* (prepared for the Canadian Council on Learning's Health and Learning Knowledge Centre). Antigonish, Canada: St. Francis Xavier University. Retrieved from http://www.nald.ca/library/research/sotfr/adultlit/adultlit.pdf.

Raphael, D. (2007). Addressing health inequalities in Canada: Little attention, inadequate action, limited success. In M. O'Neill, A. Pederson, S. Dupere, and I. Rootman (Eds.), *Health promotion in Canada: Critical perspectives* (pp. 106-122). Toronto, Canada: Canadian Scholars' Press.

Raphael, D. (2008). Getting serious about the social determinants of health: New directions for public health workers. *Global Health Promotion, 15*(3), 15-20.

Ronson, B., and Rootman, I. (2009). Literacy: One of the most important determinants of health. In D. Raphael (Ed.), *Social determinants of health: Canadian perspectives* (2nd ed., pp. 170-185). Toronto, Canada: Canadian Scholars' Press.

Rootman, I. (2006). Health literacy: Where are the Canadian doctors? *Canadian Medical Association Journal, 175*(6), 606-607.

Rootman, I. (2009). Relation between literacy skills and the health of Canadians. In online *Encyclopedia of Language Development*. Retrieved from.http://www.literacyencyclopedia.ca/index.php?fa=items.showand topicId=264.

Rootman, I., Frankish, J., and Kaszap, M. (2007). Health literacy: A new frontier. In M. O'Neill, A. Peterson, S. Dupere, and I. Rootman (Eds.), *Health promotion in Canada: Critical perspectives* (pp. 61-73). Toronto, Canada: Canadian Scholar's Press.

Rootman, I., and Gordon-El-Bihbety, D. (2008). *A vision for a health literate Canada: Report of the expert panel on health literacy*. Ottawa, Canada: Canadian Public Health Association.

Rootman, I., and Ronson, B. (2005). Literacy and health research in Canada: Where have we been and where should we go? *Canadian Journal of Public Health, 96*(2), 62-77.

Shohet, L. (2004). Health and literacy: Perspectives. *Literacy and Numeracy Studies, 13*(1), 65-84.

Sihota, S., and Lennard, L. (2004). *Health literacy: Being able to make the most of health.* London, England: National Consumer Council.

Tavistock Institute and Shared Intelligence. (2009). *Evaluation of the second phase of the Skilled for Health Programme: Final evaluation report.* London, England: Authors.

Thaler, R. H., and Sunstein, C. R. (2008). *Nudge: Improving decisions about health, wealth, and happiness.* New York, NY: Penguin Books.

von Wagner, C., Knight, K., Steptoe, A., and Wardle, J. (2007). Functional health literacy and health promoting behaviour in a national sample of British adults. *Journal of Epidemiology and Public Health, 61*, 1086-1090.

Wanless, D. (2004). *Securing good health for the whole population (final report)*. London, England: HM Treasury. Available from http://webarchive.nationalarchives.gov.uk/+/http://www.hm-treasury.gov. uk/consultations_and_legislation/wanless/consult_wanless04_final.cfm.

Wharf-Higgins, J., Begoray, D. L., and MacDonald, M. (2009). A social ecological conceptual framework for understanding adolescent health literacy in the health education classroom. *American Journal of Community Psychology, 16*(4), 350-362. doi:10.1007/s10464-009-9270-8.

Weiss, B. D., Mays, M. Z., Martz, W., Castro, K. M., DeWalt, D. A., Pignone, M. P., ... Hale, F. A. (2005). Quick assessment of literacy in primary care: the newest vital sign. *Annals of Family Medicine, 3*, 514-522.

Woolf, S. H., Chan, E. C. Y., Harris, R., Sheridan, S. L., Braddock, C. H. III, Kaplan, R. M., ... Tunis, S. (2005). Promoting informed choice: Transforming health care to dispense knowledge for decision making. *Annals of Internal Medicine, 143*(4), 293-300.

World Health Organization. (1986). *Ottawa charter for health promotion.* Geneva, Switzerland: Author.

World Health Organization. (1998). *Health promotion glossary.* Geneva, Switzerland: Author.

World Health Organization. (2003). *Global strategy for infant and young child feeding.* Geneva, Switzerland: Author.

World Health Organization. (2008). 2008-2013 *Action plan for the global strategy for the prevention and control of noncommunicable diseases.* Geneva, Switzerland: Author.

Zarcadoolas, C., Pleasant, A., and Greer, D. S. (2006). *Advancing health literacy: A framework for understanding and action.* San Francisco, CA: Jossey-Bass.

Zeng, Q. T., Kogan, S., Plovnick, R. M., Crowell, J., Lacroix, E. M., and Greenes, R. A. (2004). Positive attitudes and failed queries: An exploration of the conundrums of health information retrieval. *International Journal of Medical Information, 73*, 45-55.

In: Health Literacy in Context   ISBN: 978-1-61942-921-5
Eds.: D.Begoray, D.Gillis, G.Rowlands © 2012 Nova Science Publishers, Inc.

Chapter 4

HEALTH LITERACY AND HEALTH OUTCOMES

Joanne Protheroe, Michael S. Wolf and Albert Lee*

ABSTRACT

In this chapter, we examine the impact of low health literacy on health outcomes. We review the body of research that has been published internationally, noting that the majority of these studies are describing simply the various associations between adult literacy skills and health outcomes rather than causation. Specifically, lack of reading fluency and low levels of health vocabulary (i.e., low literacy as applied to health) have been linked to problems with the use of preventive services, delayed diagnoses, understanding of one's medical condition, adherence to medical instructions, self-management skills, physical and mental health, and increased mortality risk. We consider what this evidence may say about possible causal pathways between health literacy and health outcomes and, very briefly, discuss the potential for interventions.

_____

* Corresponding author: E-mail: joanne.protheroe@keele.ac.uk.

INTRODUCTION

There are several definitions of health literacy (see Chapter 2 for full discussion) that guide researchers and practitioners. In the United States of America (US), where many of the research findings on health literacy and health outcomes have been published, health literacy has been considered a domain of general literacy that is specific to health-related activities. These researchers have commonly used the definition of health literacy adopted by the United States Institute of Medicine (US IOM), which defines it as:

> ... the degree to which individuals have the capacity to obtain, process, and understand basic health information and services needed to make appropriate health decisions. (Ratzan and Parker, 2000, as cited in Nielsen-Bohlman, Panzer, and Kindig, 2004, p. 20)

This definition can be described as a *basic skills* definition; however, the concept of health literacy can be considered more broadly, even within this definition. Being able to obtain, process or interpret, and understand information includes knowing whether to seek professional help, where to seek help, how to—*and being able to*—ask the right questions, and how to follow treatment regimes. While health literacy is not simply the ability to read, basic literacy and numeracy skills with their associated cognitive development are fundamental requirements for health literacy. This definition implies that health literacy is a set of skills or capacities that individuals require to fully participate in their health care.

The World Health Organisation (WHO, 1998) places a slightly different emphasis when it defines health literacy as:

> ... the cognitive and social skills which determine the motivation and ability of individuals to again access to, understand and use information in ways which promote and maintain good health. (WHO, p. 10)

This broader definition suggests that a health-literate individual would, in addition to the previously considered set of capacities, be *motivated* to adopt healthy behaviours and have the *self-efficacy* to complete defined tasks. However, in this chapter, the research evidence discussed relates to the IOM definition as this has been used in the majority of these studies.

As health researchers and health professionals, we are interested in the impact of health literacy on a broad range of health outcomes; therefore, we describe how health literacy has been shown to have an effect on health knowledge and self-care skills, health attitudes and beliefs, health behaviour, and global health measures. This is in line with the logic model (Figure 1) used to analyse studies for a recent systematic review of health literacy interventions and outcomes (Berkman et al., 2011).

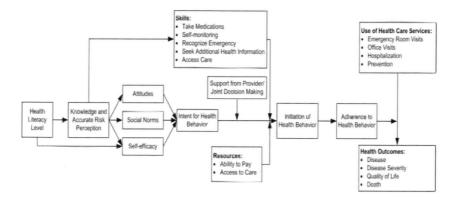

Figure 1. Logic model for analyzing studies of health literacy. From *Health Literacy Interventions and Outcomes: An Updated Systematic Review* (p. ED-3), by N. D. Berkman et al, 2011, Rockville, MD: Agency for Healthcare Research and Quality. Copyright 2011 by the AHRQ. (Document in the public domain and may be reproduced.).

What began as a handful of studies evaluating associations between poor reading ability and health knowledge and behaviours in the 1970s has expanded to an independent field of study. Currently, there are over 1,500 health literacy related publications—although a large proportion simply addresses the readability of health materials. In the US, the federal government has identified improving the health literacy of Americans in order to improve health outcomes as a priority for national public health efforts. In 2004, the United Kingdom (UK) National Consumer Council produced a document to summarise the main research evidence on health literacy (largely US based). It found that low health literacy appeared to be particularly prevalent among lower socioeconomic groups, ethnic minorities, the elderly, and those with chronic conditions or disabilities (Sihota and Lennard, 2004). As there has been little research into health literacy in the UK, most of the available evidence quoted in this chapter comes from research conducted in the US and Canada.

The concept of health literacy has continued to evolve, moving away from simply examining health literacy from the perspective of an individual patient and his or her skill set to consider the interaction between individual capacities, the health care system, and the broader society. Consequently, the measurement of health literacy at the individual level is clearly inadequate (Baker, 2006). For example, in long-term condition management, self-efficacy, greater understanding of the benefits of different health actions, personal health skills in adopting certain specific behaviours, self-monitoring, and family support are all important factors leading to better clinical outcomes, alongside the interaction with the health care system. In addition to being inadequate to measure health literacy at a purely individual level, measures that have been used at an individual level are themselves limited. The two measures that have been commonly used in the literature referred to later in this chapter are the Rapid Estimate of Adult Literacy in Medicine (REALM; Davis et al., 1993) and the Test of Functional Health Literacy in Adults (TOFHLA; Parker et al. 1995). REALM is a test of word recognition and pronunciation; TOFHLA also tests literacy and some comprehension. Neither measure fully encompasses the broad range of skills and capacities referred to in most definitions; however, they have the advantage of being relatively easy to include as an outcome measure in a research study.

In this chapter, we review the body of research describing health literacy and health outcomes; however, these studies describe more simply the various associations between adult literacy skills and health outcomes. Specifically, brief measures of reading fluency and health vocabulary have been linked to problems with the use of preventive services, delayed diagnoses, understanding of one's medical condition, adherence to medical instructions, self-management skills, physical and mental health, and increased mortality risk. The nature of these relationships will be examined in detail and likely causal pathways discussed.

A SUMMARY OF CURRENT RESEARCH EVIDENCE

While much of the published evidence is from the US and Canada, we have attempted, where possible to include international data. Before we present research evidence relating to the impact of health literacy on health outcomes, it is important to describe the prevalence of low health literacy; we present estimates of the extent of the problem from the UK, US, Canada, and Australia.

Multiple studies in the US and Canada have shown that many patients have limited ability to understand written health information. Slightly less than a fifth (19%) of the US adult population performs at the lowest health literacy levels, indicating difficulty using relatively simple texts; of these, 7% are estimated to be unable to perform even simple tasks with a high degree of proficiency (Rudd, 2007). The Canadian Council on Learning (CCL, 2008) reported that the majority of adult Canadians aged 16 and over (60%) do not have the necessary skills to manage their health adequately. Similar rates (59%) have been reported in Australia (Australian Bureau of Statistics, 2006). In the 2003 Skills for Life survey undertaken by the Department for Education and Skills in England (DES, 2003), 46% of people scored below the level of general literacy needed to achieve their full potential with 3% at the most basic level (i.e., illiterate); the results indicated even worse figures of 75% and 5%, respectively, for numeracy. This must impact all levels of health knowledge and empowerment, including ethical issues such as achieving fully informed consent for medical procedures. The remainder of the research evidence presented in this chapter is organised into sections in line with the logic model of health literacy shown in Figure 1.

Health Knowledge and Self-Care Skills

Some of the earliest evidence linking low health literacy to health outcomes relates to poorer health knowledge (Berkman et al., 2011). There is evidence that individuals with limited health literacy possess less health knowledge and, consequently, have poorer self-management skills. Williams, Baker, Honig, Lee, and Nowlan (1998) interviewed patients presenting to an urban hospital asthma clinic and/or emergency department and found those with low health literacy had poorer asthma knowledge. In a similar study, less literate patients with hypertension and diabetes were also reported to have poorer knowledge of these conditions (Williams, Baker, Parker, and Nurss, 1998) Other research studies have since confirmed this relationship in a multitude of contexts. Among individuals living with HIV/AIDS, those with limited literacy were less able to explain or define commonly used terms in their illness management (e.g., CD4 lymphocyte count and viral load) and to identify antiviral medications in their regimen even with the aid of pictures (Kalichman and Rompa, 2000; Wolf et al., 2004).

A great deal of attention has highlighted the association between low health literacy and treatment misunderstanding, including medication names, indications, and instructions. Davis et al. (2006) conducted a multisite study among adults and found those with limited literacy had higher rates of misunderstanding directions for using their medications that were provided by either the physician or pharmacist; the problem extended to icons used for medication warnings and precautions. Finally, in perhaps one of the most indicting studies linking literacy skills to medical understanding, Gazmararian, Williams, Peel, and Baker (2003) interviewed patients with asthma, hypertension, diabetes, or congestive heart failure and found that low health literacy was an independent predictor of poor knowledge across all of the studied chronic conditions.

Much of the difficulty patients have in understanding written health information results from a general problem with reading fluency. In addition, many patients have extremely limited background knowledge of how their body works and common health conditions. Not everyone has had the opportunity to study biology or even basic science at school. Without this background knowledge, it is often very difficult for patients to understand new information given to them by their doctors and health care team, whether it is written or spoken. Doctors and other health care providers frequently use words that are unfamiliar to patients; they also present conceptual information that is so unfamiliar that it does not make sense, even if said simply. For example, when explaining what a range of normal fasting blood sugar is to patients with diabetes, research has shown that many patients did not even realize that there is sugar in their blood (D. W. Baker, personal communication, July 2009).

Attitudes and Beliefs

Another impact of low health literacy and a barrier to effective understanding of health and health care may be divergent health beliefs (see Chapter 6). Patients and doctors may have widely divergent beliefs about health and illness. Lay health beliefs are those views held by members of society who are not health professionals. For health professionals, medical training has led to an emphasis on formal biomedical and epidemiological approaches to understanding health behaviour. These differing perspectives between professionals and patients relate not only to their personal beliefs about health and illness but also to their expectations of medical care, their priorities for treatment, and the ways in which they interpret information about disease (Carr and Donovan, 1998). These health beliefs, which diverge from those of their health care provider, may be mediated or exacerbated by low health literacy; and the possible stigmatisation of low literacy may prevent patients from asking for clarification (Parikh, Parker, Nurss, Baker, and

Williams, 1996). For example, terms used for routine tests and commonly used phrases for medical interventions may be interpreted differently; different expectations of medical care may lead to women viewing baby health checks not as helpful health promotion and prevention but as a morality check up that the doctor is examining the child for signs of abuse (Hodgins, Millar, and Barry, 2006). Patients' attitudes and beliefs may be influenced by their culture and the community with which they identify themselves (see Chapter 6). A lack of awareness and sensitivity—and possibly low health literacy—in health professionals may serve to exacerbate these differences.

Health Behaviours

In the logic model (Figure 1), knowledge, skills, and attitudes all have an impact on health behaviours. In the literature, patients with low health literacy have been shown to demonstrate poor access and utilisation of health services with both decreased use of preventative services and greater use of emergency services (Berkman et al., 2011). Scott, Gazmararian, Williams, and Baker (2002) found individuals with low health literacy to be less likely to have received an influenza or pneumococcal vaccination, mammogram, or cervical smear, if eligible. Dolan and Frisina (2002) found that low literacy was significantly associated with poor knowledge and negative attitudes toward use of colon cancer screening tests. Earlier Davis et al. (1996) had found that knowledge, attitudes, and screening intention for mammography were strongly associated with literacy skills in a group of screening-eligible women. A recent study (Chow et al., 2010) of Asian women assessing their knowledge and attitudes toward cervical cancer, common in both Asian and Western countries, revealed that 58% of respondents professed to know quite a lot about it and only 19% had heard of human papilloma virus; these results reflect a low level of health literacy for a disease that is preventable but potentially life threatening. Bennett et al. (1998) reported that racial disparities in advanced stage presentation of prostate cancer were partly explained by lower literacy levels among African-Americans, suggesting that low literacy may be associated with late or less frequent screening. These findings were confirmed using more recent data where a blood test to measure prostatic specific antigen is widely used for determining the extent of disease at time of diagnosis (Wolf et al., 2006).

Williams et al. (1998) evaluated asthma patients' technique for using a metered dose inhaler; those with low health literacy skills were less able to demonstrate proper inhaler technique compared to those with adequate literacy. Three additional studies found that individuals with limited health literacy reported poorer medication adherence compared to those with adequate health literacy (Gazmararian et al., 2006; Kalichman, Graham, Luke, and Austin, 2002; Wolf et al., 2007). Schillinger et al. (2002) found that among diabetic patients those with low health literacy skills were less able to achieve tight glycaemic control and reported higher rates of retinopathy as the result of poor diabetes self-care. In a randomized control study among Chinese diabetic patients in Hong Kong, patients who received an intensive health literacy intervention (based on self-management skills) had significantly improved eating habits at follow-up (Lee et al., 2011).

Finally, in a survey of British adults, an increase in health literacy was associated with an increased likelihood to adopt healthy behaviours (e.g., eating the recommended five portions of fruit and vegetables, not smoking) and having good self-rated health. This was independent of age, education, gender, ethnicity, and income (von Wagner, Knight, Steptoe, and Wardle, 2007). These findings are supported by an updated systematic review of health literacy interventions and outcomes, which stated that:

> Differences in health literacy level were consistently associated with increased hospitalizations, greater emergency care use, lower use of mammography, lower receipt of influenza vaccine, poorer ability to demonstrate taking medications appropriately, poorer ability to interpret labels and health messages, and, among seniors, poorer overall health status and higher mortality. Health literacy level potentially mediates disparities between blacks and whites. (Berkman et al., 2011, p. v)

Health Status

Individuals with limited health literacy report experiencing poorer health. Baker, Parker, Williams, and Clark (1998) examined the relationship between health literacy and self-reported health among patients presenting to the emergency department or ambulatory clinic at one of two urban public hospitals. Patients with low health literacy were more than twice as likely to self-report poor health on a single-item question, even after adjusting for age, gender, race, and markers of economic deprivation. Similar findings were reported in the UK Skilled for Life survey (DES, 2003); of those who described themselves as having poor or very poor health, 37% had low literacy skills compared with 24% who had adequate literacy. Research has indicated that self-reported health status appears to be a relatively good predictor of health outcomes (Benjamins, Hummer, Eberstein, and Nam, 2004); and the International Adult Literacy and Skills Survey indicated a link between literacy, health literacy, and self-reported health.

Canadians with the lowest health literacy scores are 2.5 times as likely to see themselves as being in fair or poor health as those with high health literacy scores; this relationship holds even after removing the impact of age, gender, education, mother tongue, immigration, and Aboriginal status (Canadian Council on Learning, 2008). Wolf, Gazmararian, and Baker (2005) investigated the relationship between inadequate health literacy and self-reported functional health status among older adults. Those with low health literacy had a higher prevalence of diabetes and congestive heart failure; they reported worse physical and mental health, greater difficulty with activities of daily living, and limitations due to physical health. Likewise, Mancuso and Rincon (2006) reported that among adult asthma patients limited health literacy was associated with poorer physical health, worse quality of life, and a greater number of emergency department visits. Previously, two studies by Baker (1999) and colleagues (Baker et al., 2002) reported that patients with inadequate health literacy had a greater risk of hospital admission compared to those with adequate literacy. A diabetic self-care programme, aiming to improve self efficacy, showed a marked improvement in diabetic self-efficacy and body mass index and an improvement in the proportion of normal glycaemic control (Lee et al., 2011).

Research has identified low health literacy as a significant risk factor to greater mortality. Sudore et al. (2006) found in over 2,500 black and white elders that low health literacy was associated with a 75% increased risk for all-cause mortality compared to those with adequate health literacy. Similarly, Baker et al. (2007) found low health literacy to be significantly and independently associated with a 51% greater mortality risk; the association was found to be significant for cardiovascular causes but not for cancer.

Numeracy and Health Outcomes

Numeracy is an important—and often underrepresented in research—component of health literacy. Skills in numeracy are important in understanding quantitative health information, such as risk information, or in understanding a complex medication regime; they are a key component in effective self-management of chronic diseases such as diabetes (Osborn, Cavanaugh, Wallston, White, and Rothman, 2009). There has been limited research examining the effect of numeracy per se on health outcomes. Berkman et al. (2011) reported that the strength of evidence of numeracy studies is low, limiting conclusions regarding numeracy and health outcomes. However, two studies did suggest that numeracy levels may be the mediator in health disparities. Osborn et al. (2009) examined whether health literacy, general numeracy, and diabetes-related numeracy could explain the association between African Americans and poor glycaemic control in patients with diabetes; they found that diabetes-related numeracy, not race, was significantly related to poor glycaemic control. In a study of health literacy, numeracy, and patients' ability to manage a mock HIV medication regime, Waldrop-Valverde et al. (2009) found that women appeared to be significantly less able than men to manage and that these results were mediated by numeracy skills.

EXTENT AND NATURE OF ASSOCIATIONS

While the relationship between health literacy and health outcomes is not entirely clear, there are plausible mechanisms by which literacy could directly affect health behaviours, compliance with medications, and other pathways to health (Baker, 1999; DeWalt, Berkman, Sheridan, Lohr, and Pignone, 2004; Paasche-Orlow and Wolf, 2007). Empirical data collected over the past two decades support these links. As we have described, limited health literacy has been associated with less health knowledge (Gazmararian et al., 2003), worse self-management skills (Schillinger et al., 2002), higher hospitalization rates, (Baker et al., 1998, 2002; Rudd, 2007), poorer health (Wolf et al., 2005), and greater mortality (Baker et al., 2007; Sudore et al., 2006). Literacy is more strongly associated with these outcomes than years of education (Baker et al., 2002, 2007; Wolf et al., 2005; Yen and Moss, 1999). This review of the evidence suggests health literacy to be one of the strongest known socioeconomic indicators of health outcomes.

One possible causal mechanism linking lower literacy to health outcomes could be that the quality of peoples' health care experience may be compromised due to ineffective communication within the medical encounter. This is compounded by a lack of accessible health information resources to supplement what was or was not understood during the physician–patient encounter. For example, physicians often do not communicate at a level that is understood by patients with lower literacy skills nor are written materials at an appropriate reading level (Davis, Michielutte, Askov, Williams, and Weiss, 1998; Lindau, Tomori, McCarville, and Bennett, 2001). The majority of patient education materials that are distributed in physicians' offices or other health-related settings have repeatedly been found to be too complex, written at too high a level, or not organized from the patient's perspective (Davis et al., 1996; Hearth-Holmes et al., 1997; Zion and Aiman, 1989). Yet, patients with limited literacy may feel shame as a result of their poor reading ability, not understand terms used by the physician, and consequently lack the self-efficacy to seek clarification or acquire information elsewhere (Parikh et al., 1996).

In the sections above, we have presented evidence that patients with low health literacy possess less health knowledge and are more likely to hold divergent lay health beliefs—both of which could be mediating factors between low health literacy and the poorer health outcomes that are reported. Over time, these factors can contribute to worse health status as a result of inadequate use of preventive services, negative health behaviours, and poorer self-management of acquired illness. These are in line with the logic model (Figure 1).

However, health literacy can be considered not simply in terms of knowledge transfer but as capacity building. It needs to go beyond individual capacity to community development so that individuals will interact with the health care system and the broader society to build up their capacity for better health. Actions such as health communication, capacity development, community development, organization development, and policy address the issues of health literacy; education, early childhood development, living and working conditions, and culture are possible determinants of health literacy (Rootman and Ronson, 2005).

CONCLUSION

On an individual patient level, limited health literacy is a serious barrier to communication in health care and may affect individuals' ability to manage their health. On a wider scale, there is evidence that limited health literacy is implicated as an important social determinant of health (Marmot, 2010). Policy makers, patient educators, and clinicians should include the development and implementation of new strategies to address raising population health literacy as an important goal. It is difficult to draw firm conclusions about effective strategies and interventions to improve health literacy from the research evidence because the quality of studies undertaken and the variety of outcome measures used in studies has been mixed (Berkman et al., 2011). However, some understanding can be drawn from the range of experience and evidence accruing; and some broad guidance for the development of health literacy interventions, ranging from those directed at the individual level through to those aimed for group and population-based delivery, can be offered. Key components of effective interventions described in the recent systematic review by Berkman et al. (2011) were their high intensity, theory basis, pilot testing before implementation, emphasis on skill building, and delivery of the intervention by a health professional (e.g., pharmacist, diabetes educator).

Clinicians and other health professionals should seek to communicate orally with all patients in a clear and concise manner and to provide easy-to-understand print and visual materials to reinforce health messages. For example, one technique frequently used by clinicians to check understanding and recall of the consultation is to ask patients to repeat critical information in their own words. Using this technique—*teach back*—clearly establishes that the patient has understood the consultation. By closing the communication loop in this way, clinicians can identify which explanations patients most often understand. Utilizing the teach-back technique and guided imagery during clinical encounters as well as incorporating adult education design standards into the creation of health materials will promote the effective transfer of information between health care providers and patients.

As health care becomes increasingly complex with new technologies and cost restraints, problems will become even more apparent with greater burdens placed on patients when attempting to access health services and navigate complex health care systems (Wolf and Schorling, 2000). Policy makers, patient educators, and clinicians must continue to (a) strive to increase the health literacy of individuals and families and empower all to better understand their health and self-care roles and (b) take action on health information for the benefit of their own physical and mental wellbeing.

Questions for Reflection

1)   What are the desirable health impacts and health outcomes that we would expect to observe with improvement of patients' health literacy? Do we want to focus on changing attitudes, improving self-

efficacy, behavioural modification, changes of health status, or changes of clinical parameters? Why?

2) Should we move toward empowering the community by improving health literacy to create a more supportive environment for health and creating a social norm for healthy behaviours? What might be the benefits/challenges of such an approach? What is the role of health literacy in creating more supportive environments for health and creating a social norm for healthy behaviours?

3) Should we consider health literacy as capacity building for self-care and self-management in long-term illnesses?

4) Would improvement of health literacy lead to de-professionalisation of health care professionals? Is this an important problem for you and for society at large?

5) Would improvement of health literacy of the general population lead to increased demand of health service utilisation with enhancement of capacity to understand complex health issues? How might other demands be reduced?

6) Should effective health communication become an integral component of health literacy? How might this be achieved? How can practitioners become more effective in communicating with their patients about the health consequences of their decisions and actions?

7) Is there enough evidence to support that health literacy is an important determinant of health? What steps need to be taken to strengthen the evidence linking health literacy to health outcomes?

8) Are health professionals health literate?

ACKNOWLEDGMENTS

The authors would like to acknowledge contributions to this chapter from David Baker, Stacey Bailey, and Kirsten McCaffery.

REFERENCES

Australian Bureau of Statistics. (2006). *Health literacy, Australia*. Canberra, Australia: Author.

Baker, D. W. (1999). Reading between the lines: Deciphering the connections between literacy and health. *Journal of General Internal Medicine, 14,* 315-317.

Baker, D. W. (2006). The meaning and the measure of health literacy. *Journal of General Internal Medicine, 21*(8), 878-883. doi:10.1111/j.1525-1497.2006.00540.x

Baker, D. W., Gazmararian, J. A., Williams, M. V., Scott, T., Parker, R. M., Green, D., ... Peel, J. (2002). Functional health literacy and the risk of hospital admission among Medicare managed care enrollees. *American Journal of Public Health, 92*(8), 1278-1283.

Baker, D. W., Parker, R. M., Williams, M. V., and Clark, W. S. (1998). Health literacy and the risk of hospital admission. *Journal of General Internal Medicine, 13,* 791-798.

Baker, D. W., Wolf, M. S., Feinglass, J., Thompson, J. A., Gazmararian, J. A., and Huang, J. (2007). Health literacy and mortality among elderly persons. *Archives of Internal Medicine, 167*(14), 1503-1509. doi:<p>10.1001/archinte.167.14.1503</p>

Benjamins, M. R., Hummer, R. A., Eberstein, I. W., and Nam, C. B. (2004). Self-reported health and adult mortality risk: An analysis of cause-specific mortality. *Social Science and Medicine, 59,* 1297-1306.

Bennett, C. L., Ferreira, M. R., Davis, T. C., Kaplan, J., Weinberger, M., Kuzel, T., ... Sartor, O. (1998). Relation between literacy, race, and stage of presentation among low-income patients with prostate cancer. *Journal of Clinical Oncology, 16,* 3101-3104.

Berkman, N. D., Sheridan, S. L., Donahue, K. E., Halpern, D. J., Viera, A., Crotty, K., ... Viswanathan, M. (2011). *Health literacy interventions and outcomes: An updated systematic review* (Evidence Report/Technology Assessment No. 199; AHRQ Publication No. 11-E006). Rockville, MD: Agency for Healthcare Research and Quality.

Canadian Council on Learning. (2008). *Health literacy in Canada: A healthy understanding.* Ottawa, Canada: Author.

Carr, A. J., and Donovan, J. L. (1998). Why doctors and patients disagree. *British Journal of Rheumatology, 37,* 1-4.

Chow, S. N., Soon, R., Park, J. S., Pancharoen, C., Qiao, Y. L., Basu, P., and Ngan, H. Y. S. (2010). Knowledge, attitudes, and communication around human papillomavirus (HPV) vaccination amongst urban Asian mothers and physicians. *Vaccine, 28*(22), 3809-3817.

Davis, T. C., Arnold, C., Berkel, H. J., Nandy, I., Jackson, R. H., and Glass, J. (1996). Knowledge and attitude on screening mammography among low-literate, low-income women. *Cancer, 78,* 1912-1920.

Davis, T. C., Long, S. W., Jackson, R. H., Mayeaux, E. J., George, R. B., Murphy, P. W., and Crouch, M. A. (1993). Rapid estimate of adult literacy in medicine: A shortened screening instrument. *Family Medicine, 25,* 391-395.

Davis, T. C., Michielutte, R., Askov, E. N., Williams, M. V., and Weiss, B. D. (1998). Practical assessment of adult literacy in health care. *Health Education and Behavior, 25,* 613-624.

Davis, T. C., Wolf, M. S., Bass, P. F., III, Thompson, J. A., Tilson, H. H., Neuberger, M., and Parker, R. M. (2006). Literacy and misunderstanding prescription drug labels. *Annals of Internal Medicine, 145,* 887-894.

DeWalt, D. A., Berkman, N. D., Sheridan, S., Lohr, K. N., and Pignone, M. P. (2004). Literacy and health outcomes: A systematic review of the literature. *Journal of General Internal Medicine, 19*(12), 1228-1239.

Dolan, J. G., and Frisina, S. (2002). Randomized controlled trial of a patient decision aid for colorectal cancer screening. *Medical Decision Making, 22,* 125-139.

Gazmararian, J. A., Kripalani, S., Miller, M. J., Echt, K. V., Ren, J., and Rask, K. (2006). Factors associated with medication refill adherence in cardiovascular-related diseases: A focus on health literacy. *Journal of General Internal Medicine, 21,* 1215-1221.

Gazmararian, J. A., Williams, M. V., Peel, J., and Baker, D. W. (2003). Health literacy and knowledge of chronic disease. *Patient Education and Counseling, 51*(3), 267-275.

Hearth-Holmes, M., Murphy, P. W., Davis, T. C., Nandy, I., Elder, C. G., Broadwell, L. H., et al. (1997). Literacy in patients with a chronic disease: Systemic lupus erythematosus and the reading level of patient education materials. *Journal of Rheumatology, 24,* 2335-2339.

Hodgins, M., Millar, M., and Barry, M. M. (2006). "...it's all the same no matter how much fruit or vegetables or fresh air we get": Traveller women's perceptions of illness causation and health inequalities. *Social Science and Medicine, 62,* 1978-1990.

Kalichman, S. C., Graham, J., Luke, W., and Austin, J. (2002). Perceptions of health care among persons living with HIV/AIDS who are not receiving antiretroviral medications. *AIDS Patient Care and STDs, 16,* 233-240.

Kalichman, S. C., and Rompa, D. (2000). Functional health literacy is associated with health status and health-related knowledge in people living with HIV-AIDS. *Journal of Acquired Immune Deficiency Syndromes, 25,* 337-344.

Lee, A., Siu, C. F., Leung, K. T., Lau, L. C., Chan, C. C., and Wong, K. K. (2011). General practice and social service partnership for better clinical outcomes, patient self efficacy and lifestyle behaviours of diabetic care: Randomised control trial of a chronic care model. *Postgraduate Medical Journal, 87,* 688-693.

Lindau, S. T., Tomori, C., McCarville, M. A., and Bennett, C. L. (2001). Improving rates of cervical cancer screening and Pap smear follow-up for low-income women with limited health literacy. *Cancer Investigation, 19,* 316-323.

Mancuso, C. A., and Rincon, M. (2006). Impact of health literacy on longitudinal asthma outcomes. *Journal of General Internal Medicine, 21,* 813-817.

Marmot, M. (2010). *Fair society, healthy lives: Strategic review of health inequalities in England post-2010.* London, England: The Marmot Review Team. Retrieved from www.marmotreview.org.

Nielsen-Bohlman, L., Panzer, A. M., and Kindig, D. A. (Eds.). (2004). *Health literacy: A prescription to end confusion.* Washington, DC: Institute of Medicine of the National Academies and The National Academies Press.

Osborn, C. Y., Cavanaugh, K., Wallston, K. A., White, R. O., and Rothman, R. L. (2009). Diabetes numeracy: An overlooked factor in understanding racial disparities in glycemic control. *Diabetes Care, 32,* 1614-1619.

Paasche-Orlow, M. K., and Wolf, M. S. (2007). The causal pathways linking health literacy to health outcomes. *American Journal of Health Behavior, 31*(S1), S19-26.

Parikh, N. S., Parker, R. M., Nurss, J. R., Baker, D. W., and Williams, M. V. (1996). Shame and health literacy: The unspoken connection. *Patient Education and Counseling, 27*(1), 33-39.

Parker, R. M., Baker, D. W., Williams, M. V., and Nurss, J. R. (1995). The test of functional health literacy in adults: A new instrument for measuring patients' literacy skills. *Journal of General Internal Medicine, 10,* 537-541.

Ratzan, S. C., and Parker, R. M. (2000). Introduction. In *National library of medicine current bibliographies in medicine: Health literacy* (NLM Pub. No. CBM 2000-1); C. R. Sedlen, M. Zorn, S. C. Ratzan, and N. Lurie (Eds.). Bethesda, MD: National Institutes of Health, US Department of Health and Human Services.

Rootman, I., and Ronson, B. (2005). Literacy and health research in Canada: Where have we been and where should we go? *Canadian Journal of Public Health, 96*(S2), S62-77.

Rudd, R. E. (2007). Health literacy skills of U.S. adults. *American Journal of Health Behavior, 31*(S1), S8-18.

Schillinger, D., Grumbach, K., Piette, J., Wang, F., Osmond, D., Daher, C., ... Bindman, A. B. (2002). Association of health literacy with diabetes outcomes. *Journal of the American Medical Association, 288*(4), 475-482.

Scott, T. L., Gazmararian, J. A., Williams, M. V., and Baker, D. W. (2002). Health literacy and preventive health care use among Medicare enrollees in a managed care organization. *Medical Care, 40*(5), 395-404.

Sihota, S., and Lennard, L. (2004). *Health literacy: Being able to make the most of health.* London, England: National Consumer Council.

Sudore, R. L., Yaffe, K., Satterfield, S., Harris, T. B., Mehta, K. M., Simonsick, E. M., ... Schillinger, D. (2006). Limited literacy and mortality in the elderly: The health, aging, and body composition study. *Journal of General Internal Medicine, 21*(8), 806-812.

United Kingdom Department for Education and Skills. (2003). *The skills for life survey: A national needs and impact survey of literacy, numeracy and ICT skills.* London, England: Author.

von Wagner, C., Knight, K., Steptoe, A., and Wardle, J. (2007). Functional health literacy and health promoting behaviour in a national sample of British adults. *Journal of Epidemiology and Community Health, 61,* 1086-1090.

Waldrop-Valverde, D., Jones, D. L., Jayaweera, D., Gonzalez, P., Romero, J., and Ownby, R. L. (2009). Gender differences in medication management capacity in HIV infection: The role of health literacy and numeracy. *AIDS and Behavior, 13,* 46-52.

Williams, M. V., Baker, D. W., Honig, E. G., Lee, T. M., and Nowlan, A. (1998). Inadequate literacy is a barrier to asthma knowledge and self-care. *Chest, 114,* 1008-1015.

Williams, M. V., Baker, D. W., Parker, R. M., and Nurss, J. R. (1998). Relationship of functional health literacy to patients' knowledge of their chronic disease. A study of patients with hypertension and diabetes. *Archives of Internal Medicine, 158,* 166-172.

Wolf, M. S., Davis, T. C., Cross, J. T., Marin, E., Green, K., and Bennett, C. L. (2004). Health literacy and patient knowledge in a Southern US HIV clinic. *International Journal of STD and AIDS, 15,* 747-752.

Wolf, M. S., Davis, T. C., Osborn, C. Y., Skripkauskas, S., Bennett, C. L., and Makoul, G. (2007). Literacy, self-efficacy, and HIV medication adherence. *Patient Education and Counseling, 65,* 253-260.

Wolf, M. S., Gazmararian, J. A., and Baker, D. W. (2005). Health literacy and functional health status among older adults. *Archives of Internal Medicine, 165,* 1946-1952.

Wolf, M. S., Knight, S. J., Lyons, E. A., Durazo-Arvizu, R., Pickard, S. A., Arseven, A., ... Bennett, C. L. (2006). Literacy, race, and PSA level among low-income men newly diagnosed with prostate cancer. *Urology, 68*(1), 89-93.

Wolf, A. M., and Schorling, J. B. (2000). Does informed consent alter elderly patients' preferences for colorectal cancer screening? Results of a randomized trial. *Journal of General Internal Medicine, 15,* 24-30.

World Health Organization. (1998). *Health promotion glossary.* Geneva, Switzerland: Author.

Yen, I. H., and Moss, N. (1999). Unbundling education: A critical discussion of what education confers and how it lowers risk for disease and death. *Annals of the New York Academy of Sciences, 896,* 350-351.

Zion, A. B., and Aiman, J. (1989). Level of reading difficulty in the American College of Obstetricians and Gynecologists patient education pamphlets. *Obstetrics and Gynecology, 74,* 955-960.

In: Health Literacy in Context   ISBN: 978-1-61942-921-5
Eds.: D.Begoray, D.Gillis, G.Rowlands © 2012 Nova Science Publishers, Inc.

Chapter 5

HEALTH LITERACY AND LIFELONG LEARNING

Deborah L. Begoray, E. Anne Marshall, Laura P. Shone and Gillian Rowlands*

ABSTRACT

Health literacy is important throughout life and is, therefore, a crucial goal for lifelong learning both within and beyond formal educational settings. In turn, more educational involvement throughout life is correlated with an increase in health literacy, including the emerging concept of mental health literacy, and healthy behaviours. The basis for adult learning behaviours begins to be established in childhood and adolescence; however, learning through adulthood has a vitally important influence on health. Critical health literacy and empowerment arise from knowledge and skills in dealing proactively with health information. One promising example program, *Skilled for Health*, demonstrates various elements of health literacy and lifelong learning. Seniors who continue to engage in learning activities also improve their health. More research in lifelong learning and health literacy impact needs to include investigations of technology, especially as used by the commercial media and on the Internet; more research with adolescents; better measurement tools; knowledge translation (converting theoretical knowledge to

---

* Corresponding author: E-mail: dbegoray@uvic.ca.

practical application); and a more detailed understanding of mental health literacy.

INTRODUCTION

Health literacy and lifelong learning are closely related. In this chapter, we make the case that health literacy is an important goal for lifelong learning and that, in turn, greater educational involvement throughout life is correlated to an increase in health literacy and healthy behaviours. We base our argument on principles of health promotion and lifelong learning.

We contend that health literacy is an outcome of health education and can, as such, contribute to health. Health in this case is a holistic concept, including physical, emotional, spiritual, and mental wellness. Health literacy skills are learned and practiced in a variety of formal and informal settings—what has sometimes been called life-wide learning (Field, 2005).

We begin with an overview of health and health literacy. We next discuss learning in general and lifelong learning in particular. Lifelong learning has its roots in childhood and adolescence which, in turn, leads to adults choosing to continue the learning process (or not). We then outline the importance of health to the continuing positive development of individuals and communities and, more specifically, the importance of health literacy at every stage of life. We begin with the roots of adult learning behaviours as they are set in childhood and adolescence. We then examine adult learning and continuing lifelong learning in seniors. We describe one promising program, *Skilled for Health*, for the various elements of health literacy and lifelong learning. The chapter concludes with recommendations for future research and practice.

HEALTH AND HEALTH LITERACY

Health, according to the World Health Organization (WHO, 1948), is "a state of complete physical, mental and social well-being and not merely the absence of disease or infirmity" (p. 1). How health is achieved and maintained is a major concern for individuals, communities, governmental, and nongovernmental agencies worldwide. Health literacy, we suggest, is a key contributor to health and an outcome of health education and lifelong learning participation.

In this chapter, our definition (for other definitions, see Chapter 2) of health literacy is "the ability to access, understand, evaluate and communicate information as a way to promote, maintain and improve health in a variety of settings across the life-course" (Rootman and Gordon-El-Bihbety, 2008, p. 3). Literacy then, according to the Organisation for Economic Co-operation and Development and Statistics Canada (1995), is "using printed and written information to function in society, to achieve one's goals and to develop one's knowledge and potential" (p. 14). We are also aware, however, that more current definitions of literacy have broadened its traditional print-based conception and basis in reading and writing. Many scholars now see that there are multiple literacies, including visual and oral literacies, and that literacy is influenced by social interactions that are a part of health literacy as well (Chinn, 2011; New London Group, 1996).

Definitions that highlight the personal growth, development, and empowerment purposes of lifelong learning (Kendall, 2005) are conceptually compatible with and comparable to WHO's (1998) often-cited definition of health promotion—"the process of enabling people to increase control over, and to improve, their health" (para.1). Implicit in this latter definition is that one's sense of control arises from more knowledge, improved skills, or better living conditions. In critiquing the narrow clinical definition of health literacy that emerged from the medical field, Nutbeam (2000) reinforced the importance of literacy in stating that "health literacy means more than being able to read pamphlets and successfully make appointments. By improving people's access to health information and their capacity to use it effectively, health literacy is critical to empowerment" (p. 264). In fact, Nutbeam's (2008) most advanced level of health literacy, critical literacy, is deemed necessary for people to "exert greater control over life events and situations" (p. 2075), connecting us once again to this central principle of health promotion through empowerment (Tones, 2002) and a lifelong journey to achieve and maintain health. Health literacy in this case is an asset that results in a better life for individuals and, therefore, for society at large (Nutbeam, 2008).

Mental health literacy is an emerging concept. It is not as well developed or researched as general health literacy but is important because it addresses the mental and emotional aspects of the 1948 WHO definition of health. WHO (2010) defined mental health as "a state of well-being in which an individual realizes his or her own abilities, can cope with the normal stresses of life, can work productively and is able to make a contribution to his or her community" (para. 7). The social and developmental aspects of mental health are clearly addressed in this definition—context is key to understanding and promoting optimal mental health. For example, a mental health priority for a North American rural adolescent girl who is exploring her identity is very different from that of an urban immigrant mother of six who is working two jobs to make ends meet.

Jorm et al. (1997) first introduced the term *mental health literacy*; they defined it as the "knowledge and beliefs about mental disorders which aid their recognition, management or prevention" (p. 182). More recently, the Canadian Alliance on Mental Illness and Mental Health (2008) proposed a broader definition of mental health literacy as "the knowledge and skills that enable people to access, understand and apply information for mental health" (p. 2). This definition emphasizes empowerment and informed decision making, a key concept in health promotion and health literacy generally.

Research supports these ideas. In the United Kingdom (UK) for example, investigators found that funded lifelong learning enhances mental health service users' adaptability (Griffiths, 2009) and that individualized lifelong learning leads to protection and recovery from mental health problems (Hammond, 2004). Differences over definitions of mental health literacy remain, however; this controversy will continue to influence research and practice in the field of mental health interventions.

LIFELONG LEARNING

Learning is holistic (i.e., having mental, physical, spiritual, and emotional aspects), occurs in developmental stages, and is constructed by individuals largely in interaction with others. This framework is one of social constructivism, first proposed by educational theorists such as Vygotsky (1978). The Canadian Council on Learning (CCL; 2009b) stated that "[l]earning plays a critical role in enabling Canadian adults to maintain the skills and knowledge needed to make informed decisions and lead successful lives" (p. 6).

While the enterprise of education is often thought of as primarily the purview of schools, we believe that people learn about health in a variety of contexts and settings. Some of these learning environments are more formal, such as the classroom; however, people are arguably more influenced by informal than formal knowledge sources. Knowledge sources may include family, friends, doctors, nurses, and government websites—all are motivated to provide supportive, accurate, and crucial information—while other knowledge sources, such as corporations, are overwhelmingly motivated by profit. In the UK however, commercial interests and government are currently jointly involved in a 'nudge' approach to improving public health, which makes it more difficult for consumers to discern what might be the best choice for their own health (Rayner and Lang, 2011). Putative health knowledge sources seek to persuade people to purchase goods and services primarily to accrue monetary benefit, whether or not the consumer derives any health enhancement (Begoray, Cimon, and Wharf Higgins, 2010). In all cases, learners need to use critical health literacy (Chinn, 2011); that is, the ability to question health information.

Health education in its most positive form has been defined as "the continuum of learning, which enables people, as individuals, and as members of social structures, to voluntarily make decisions, modify behaviors and change social conditions in ways that are health enhancing" (Joint Committee on Health Education Terminology, 1991, p. 360). Lifelong learners are characterized as individuals who have "the capacity and the desire to learn and go on learning throughout life" (Crick, Broadfoot, and Claxton, 2004, p. 247). Lifelong learning is, therefore, the concept that learning occurs across the lifespan and within and beyond formal educational settings; it is no less than the development of human potential. While this chapter concentrates on lifelong learning as primarily an endeavour of adults heavily influenced by adolescent experiences, we strongly acknowledge a continuum that begins in early childhood where, "[f]rom a pathway approach, early development from conception to five years of age is widely accepted as establishing the foundation for learning, behaviour and health throughout the life cycle" (Keating and Hertzman, 1999, and McCain and Mustard, 1999, as cited in Li, Mattes, Stanley, McMurray, and Hertzman, 2009, p. 4).

Governments are interested in their adult citizenry continuing to improve their knowledge and skills as a way to sustain economic growth. In the UK for example, policy documents on learning state that literacy "[s]kills have the potential to transform lives by transforming life chances and driving social mobility. Having higher skills also enables people to play a fuller part in society, making it more cohesive, more environmentally friendly, more tolerant and more engaged" (UK Department for Business, Innovation and Skills, 2010, p. 5). Government sponsoring of programs, however, does not necessarily guarantee the most efficacious involvement of citizens. Individuals with positive experiences in lifelong learning situations have previously developed attitudes and habits of mind that enable them to extract learning from their experiences.

In their United States (US) research, Claxton and Lucas (2009) identified eight qualities necessary for lifelong learning: curiosity, courage, exploration and investigation, experimentation, imagination, reason and discipline, sociability, and reflection. *Curiosity* allows one to dig deeper, look for new interests and perspectives, and be open-minded when considering new ideas. Someone who has *courage* embraces challenge, is not afraid to say 'I don't know, let's find out,' and persists in the face of difficulty. One who is good at *exploration and investigation* is a keen observer of people, is attentive to the complexity of situations, and can find and take advantage of resources and opportunities. The quality of *experimentation* involves the desire to try new things and enjoy looking at work in progress. Those with good *imagination* can use their inner world to explore possibilities; they can run mental stimulations of tricky situations and visualize their role. Those with *discipline and reason* are able to construct and follow a precise train of thought; they can create a plan to support their learning (e.g., creating goals and deadlines). *Sociability* enables collaboration so as to share ideas, suggestions, and resources and to offer their own ideas while being open to new ones. *Reflection* is another skill of effective lifelong learners who think carefully about the content of their learning as well as their learning process. Effective lifelong learners look for explanations of difficulties that allow them to find different avenues for further learning rather than feeling helpless.

Lifelong learning happens best through supportive processes that stimulate and empower individuals to acquire all the knowledge, values, skills, and understanding they want and require through their lifetimes and to apply them with confidence, creativity, and enjoyment in all roles, circumstances, and environments (Longworth and Davies, 1996). For Field (2005), different learning contexts suggested another dimension to the concept of lifelong learning: *lifewide* learning or learning in the "many different areas of life in which people continue to acquire and create new skills and knowledge throughout their lifespan" (p. 1). The CCL (2009a) noted, "Lifelong learning is a philosophy that involves the development of knowledge, skills and values throughout all stages of a person's life—from early childhood through adulthood" (p. 2).

Cappon (2006), and others, viewed the process of learning throughout one's lifespan as having four pillars: learning to know (acquiring knowledge and mastering cognitive/analytical learning skills), learning to do (practical skills for daily living that enable one to earn a living), learning to live together (social cohesion and cooperation), and learning to be (fulfillment of the whole person, as an individual, family member, and citizen). For each pillar, we envision several health literacy examples:

- Learning to know (e.g., navigating websites, reading pill bottle labels and prescription information pamphlets, awareness of medical clinics, laboratories, and hospitals).
- Learning to do (e.g., speaking to make appointments, watching or listening to a video of a self-care technique, asking medical professionals questions before, during, and after treatments).
- Learning to live together (e.g., listening to a child to understand her health concern, forming a group to advocate for better health care access).
- Learning to be (e.g., writing a journal to maintain mental health, achieving balance in work/school/family life, seeking positive social support).

Health-literate, lifelong learners are skilled in all these dimensions, in various settings, and with a variety of resources. For example, the *Survey of Canadian Attitudes toward Learning* (CCL, 2009b) reported that Canadian adults rely on multiple sources of information to help them achieve health and well-being. Critical, questioning behaviours that result in closer attention to the reliability of sources is an important adult life skill.

LEARNING IN THE LIFESTAGES

In order to examine how health literacy develops and how to optimize positive development, we must look across the life courses: childhood and adolescence, young and middle adulthood, and seniors.

Childhood and Adolescence

Health educators are anxious to establish healthy behaviours as early in life as possible by providing information to parents and parents-to-be. Likewise, lifelong learning scholars argue that initiating lifelong habits of inquiry and creativity begins during early childhood experiences and in the early years of formal education (Kendall, 2005). Classroom instruction that motivates students to learn—often characterized by purposeful strategies of active/experiential learning, reflection, and perspective taking—can enhance orientations toward lifelong learning (Li et al., 2009; Mayhew, Wolniak, and Pascarella, 2008).

Transition to adult health care marks a pivotal point in adolescent development and health. In the US for example, government policy makers acknowledge that adolescents must prepare for adult health care, which requires patients to make independent health care decisions and learn self-care (Washington State Department of Health, 2011). Health literacy has been studied extensively among adults but not among adolescents. We do know that adolescents learn in ways that are somewhat different than children or adults.

Significant changes in emotional and cognitive functioning during adolescence have implications for health education that are unique for this population (Tylee, Haller, Graham, Churchill, and Sanci, 2007). In childhood and adolescence, health-related behaviours become established and adolescents move toward assuming more responsibility for their own health (Kolbe, 2005; Rickwood, Dean, Wilson, and Ciarrochi, 2005), which involves significant learning. Depending on their developmental level and life experience, adolescents may be unable to understand the link between their actions and the outcomes of those actions. An educational agenda must be broad enough to not only enhance adolescents' knowledge of literacy, social, and civic skills but also strengthen adolescents' motivation and commitment to lifelong learning that will enable them to practice healthy behaviours (Friedman and Hoffman-Goetz, 2008; Greenberg et al., 2003; von Wagner, Steptoe, Wolf, and Wardle, 2009).

The good news is that the period of adolescence is rich with opportunities for health learning. Teens are developing physically, socially, and cognitively while gradually increasing their autonomy in family and social relationships. Therefore, adolescence presents opportunities for modeling health skills and positive health behaviour and is an optimal time to anticipate and plan for the transition from paediatric care to autonomous self-care (Wolf et al., 2009).

On the other hand, adolescents face significant challenges to good health. Research in the US shows that even high-income youth whose parents supervise and pay for health care may have low health literacy and may be unprepared for the challenges of adult health care. Some difficulties in the transition from child to youth health care in the US include "aging out of treatment, insurance/funding, availability of care, and practice differences" (Reiss, Gibson, and Walker, 2005, p. 116). Adolescents who have limited health literacy may encounter significant barriers to health care access, use, quality, safety, and outcomes during adolescence and their transition to self-management of health care as adults.

Effective health behaviours involve the ability to plan, initiate, and undertake actions in a deliberate sequence; to persist and solve problems; to weigh risks versus benefits for different courses of action; and to understand the consequences of decisions and actions. Adolescents also have to deal with power inequalities during interactions with people in positions of authority such as health care providers, educators, and parents. In the context of lifelong learning, adolescence is a phase of development (of skills), transition (to independence) and a time to build experience (Wolf et al., 2009).

Mental health is equally as important as physical health. Adolescents must learn to deal with the influence of peers for good (support during difficult times) and for ill (bullying). Cyberbullying—defined as the "use of information and communication technologies to support deliberate, repeated, and hostile behaviour" (http://www.cyberbullying.org)—is an area of increasing concern for teens, parents, and educators. Dating relationships is another area that is frequently fraught with challenging decisions (Begoray and Banister, 2007); adolescents need to learn to deal appropriately with sexual decision making. As adolescents become adults, a different set of learning challenges awaits them.

Adults

Recent studies support a conclusion that there is a strong relationship between general literacy and health status (see Chapter 4). Weiss et al. (1994) examined relations between literacy and health status in adults in a literacy program and found that the physical health of those with extremely low reading levels was poor compared to those with higher levels. In general, it is now well established that lower literacy is associated with poorer health and, conversely, that poor health is a barrier to lifelong learning (Perrin, 1998; Ronson and Rootman, 2009).

Rootman and Edwards (2004) concluded that direct effects of low literacy on health include difficulty in finding and understanding health information, more health problems, more mistakes with medications, and more workplace accidents. Indirect effects of literacy include lower income and higher unemployment, greater stress and psychosocial vulnerability, unhealthy habits (e.g., smoking and unprotected sexual activity), more and longer hospital visits, more difficulty in using the health care system, and higher health care costs.

Hammond (2004) studied the mental health literacy and lifelong learning of 145 participants who were interviewed about the influence that learning had held for them throughout their lives. The responses included well-being, protection and recovery from health difficulties, and the ability to deal with stressful situations. Self-esteem and self-efficacy increased in most of the participants in Hammond's study. Many respondents reported that learning increased their confidence to take control of their lives and to take on more active social roles; it enhanced personal development by allowing them to view a troubling situation with a wider context and put their difficulties into a perspective in a way that made it easier for them to cope (e.g., protecting one's mental health by learning arts through which one can express negative emotions). Lifelong learning was also found to offer respondents a stronger sense of purpose and hope, particularly for succession to better jobs or future education.

ONE PROMISING PROGRAM IN HEALTH LITERACY AND LIFELONG LEARNING: *SKILLED FOR HEALTH*

In the UK, the program *Skilled for Health* (SfH) has been developed and implemented as one way to address improvement goals for both health and, through Skills for Life learning, literacy for adults.

The overall aims of SfH are:

- To contribute to reducing health inequalities by improving health among those communities which demonstrate the worst health outcomes.
- To enhance the ability of individuals within those communities to make informed decisions about health and well-being in a variety of different settings. …
- To use health improvement topics that embed Skills for Life learning as an incentive to engage and recruit individuals who do not traditionally participate in adult learning initiatives, with a view to supporting them to progressing into other learning opportunities. (ContinYou, n.d., para. 5)

The SfH program uses health as a focus for building skills. It is notable for its learner-centred and learner-led approach. While the overarching aims of the programme are set, the objectives and content of different courses are flexible and reflect the needs of the learners and the local environment.

The SfH program has been applied in a variety of settings, including within the workplace. A recent UK report highlighted the personal and economic impact of poor employee health, estimating the annual state benefit costs, additional health costs, and loss of taxes at over £60 (US$90/€70) billion (Black, 2008; see Chapter 7). Participating employers see the courses as a way of producing a healthier, happier, and hence more productive workforce as evidenced by statements: "[d]ecrease in sickness absence due to better ability of members of the workforce to manage health issues" and "a reduction in sickness absence and absenteeism and increasing productivity" (Tavistock Institute and Shared Intelligence, 2009). Another innovation was embedding some courses within state-provided services and institutions including sectors such as the armed forces, libraries, and prisons (Tavistock, 2009). One effect of both the workplace and sector delivery sites was high engagement with working-age men, a group that is not well engaged with current UK National Health Service primary care and preventative services (Porter and Fraser, 2006).

Outcomes of the *Skilled for Health* Program

A flexible, learner-centred approach such as that adopted by the SfH program tends to be highly valued by learners (SfH, n.d.) but can be, by its very nature, difficult to objectively assess in terms of measureable outcomes. Despite this, an evaluation of the program showed some remarkable impacts from the courses. Learners perceived marked increases in knowledge about diet, smoking, alcohol, exercise, and mental well-being. Learners described changes in dietary behaviour with 85% claiming to be eating more healthily, a finding supported by data showing increased fruit and vegetable consumption. Another favourable change was that 65% of participants reported an increase in exercise. Greater knowledge about the adverse effects of smoking and excess alcohol consumption are, however, less likely to convert into a positive change in behaviours. The courses did result in self-reported improvement in general literacy skills by over 80%. This was supported by objective evidence of an increase in skill levels in 47% of participants. Finally, the SfH courses were able to demonstrate building of interactive health literacy skills. These were assessed in only two sites where some improvement in interactive health literacy, specifically confidence in discussing health with health professionals, was shown in 25% and 60% of participants, respectively.

Seniors

As adults age, they encounter additional complications in learning, such as for some seniors a decline in memory (Czernochowski, Fabiani, and Friedman, 2008) or anxiety about learning using computer technology. Seniors are more often faced with long term conditions requiring interactions with a wider range of health care providers, adherence to advice on self- care and disease management, and the ability to think critically about conflicting health claims and advice encountered in media or through friends and family members.

In today's rapidly changing society and in many cultures but not all, seniors are too often not valued for their experience and wisdom but rather are seen as a drain on the public purse especially in health care (Chappell and Hollander, 2011). There is a great need for educational opportunities in later life; indeed, some scholars believe that "responding to the learning needs of older people may be one of our greatest challenges" (Cusack, 1995, p. 313).

In order to empower seniors and support them to become the leaders of lifelong learning in their community, Cusack (1995) adapted Knowles' earlier work on adult learning and used the following principles throughout her project: (a) involve the participants in the decision making of every aspect of the program; (b) follow the needs, interests, and leads of participants, instead of the needs defined by professionals; (c) give everyone equal opportunity to express their ideas; (d) use every opportunity to recognize participant's talents, contributions, and achievements; (e) recognize and build on the diversity in the group; (f) find the source of ideas; (g) encourage individuals to choose what they want to pursue and do it in their own way; and (h) encourage participants to set reasonable limits on how much they want to be involved.

Cusack (1995) trained seniors as research associates in order to conduct a needs assessment of their peers, with the goal of empowering seniors as leaders in lifelong learning. The seniors in Cusack's study reported that learning prevented them from getting depressed, resulted in mental stimulation (which many of them felt was needed in order to live a healthier life thus affecting their physical health), and increased their self-esteem and the ability to express their ideas. Taken together, these findings suggest that lifelong learning can empower and enable individuals, especially seniors, to cope with potentially difficult situations and to help them believe in themselves and their capabilities.

KEY KNOWLEDGE GAPS FOR FUTURE RESEARCH

Lifelong and life-wide learning and their relation to health literacy need additional research. Several areas for further investigation include the impact of technology on health literacy, especially as used by commercial media and the Internet; more research with adolescents; more effective measurement tools; knowledge translation (converting theoretical knowledge to practical application); and further detailed understanding of mental health literacy.

Impact of the Media and the Internet

Many, if not most, forms of information, communication, and cultural transmission today, including health information, are expressed through visual and digital forms of mass media such as television, film, magazines, and the Internet (Gonzales, Glik, Davoudi, and Ang, 2004; Gray, Klein, Noyce, Sesselberg, and Cantrill, 2005; Natharius, 2004). Researchers need to examine and incorporate preferred learning methods by new generations of students— and increasingly needed by people at all life stages.

The Internet, in particular, is the natural environment of the so-called Net generation (Alvermann, Young, Green, and Wisenbaker, 1999), called digital natives (Prensky, 2001), who were born after the advent of the World Wide Web. This segment of the population relies on the Internet daily for communicating with each other, searching out information, and for entertainment (Peattie, 2007; Rideout, Roberts, and Foehr, 2005; Statistics Canada, 2007). Furthermore, digital literacy may influence one's preferences for accessing and sharing health information (Gray et al., 2005) and how that information is processed during adolescence and adulthood.

Seniors may be particularly challenged by the use of the Internet—a world that many find bewildering, especially when added to generally low levels of health literacy in the senior population (Rootman and Gordon-el-Bihbety, 2008). As health care costs increase, in large part due to an aging population and the burden of chronic disease care, there is a proliferation of technologically mediated, self-management systems for chronic disease. Increasingly, cash-strapped governments are implementing these systems with greater emphasis placed on individual responsibility for self-care. Even in countries such as Canada, which boasts a national health care system, seniors who have a lower than average level of health literacy are the main patients expected to use technology to help manage many of their health conditions (Rootman and Gordon-el-Bihbety, 2008). Mitchell and Begoray (2010) pointed out that health literacy concerns must be addressed if Canadian seniors are to be successful with new e-health systems. More research is needed to investigate the gap between the abilities of adults as they age and the literacy demands of new health care approaches. Health care providers will need to develop as educators and advocates supporting seniors. Such lifelong learning programs need to be researched with an eye to implementation in other jurisdictions as appropriate.

Seniors certainly can maintain high levels of health literacy. In a Canadian study, Wister, Malloy-Weir, Rootman, and Desjardins (2010) discovered that health literacy in seniors was strongly associated with education level and was also correlated with seniors' use of resources (e.g., manuals, reference books, and articles) and online materials. Seniors with strong health literacy were also found to be writers of notes and emails and community volunteers. Lifelong and life-wide learning for older adults in a variety of contexts—on their own or in social groups, face to face or technologically mediated—all seem important to maintain health literacy across the life course.

Research with Adolescents

There is little we know and much we can learn about health learning and literacy in health contexts for adolescents. In order to design educational interventions to foster the development of health learning capacity and subsequent health literacy, research is needed in several domains (Manganello, 2008). These areas include factors associated with positive development of health literacy during adolescence, more and better measurement tools, predictive factors associated with level of literacy in health, development and testing of interventions to teach health literacy skills, and development of resources to support adolescents in health care settings. There is a paucity of research that explores both the influence of health education on health literacy (Manganello, 2008) and the experiences and perspectives of adolescents and teachers within the formal educational context (Simpson and Freeman, 2004).

Wharf Higgins, Begoray, and MacDonald (2009) emphasized that adolescents, like all other individuals, live in a social ecology where there is a web of relationships influencing health literacy learning. Teachers of health education certainly have an impact—but so do families, friends, coaches, commercial media, and government policies and priorities (i.e., priorities for recreational parks and nutrition standards). The influence of the media on young people is both overt (in advertising) and covert (in the models of behaviour provided by video game characters). These relationships and influences need further empirical investigation.

More Effective Measurement and Assessment Tools

There is a clear need for health literacy tests for adolescents that are theoretically sound and useful in clinical settings and also in everyday contexts, such as the ability to access and evaluate health information on the Internet. Currently, only limited measures are available. In the US, Chisholm and Buchanan (2007) completed a pilot validation of the Test of Functional Health Literacy in Adults (TOFHLA) for teens. Davis et al. (2006) sought to validate the Rapid Estimate of Adolescent Literacy in Medicine (REALM-Teen) for adolescents; however, this word-recognition test with reading comprehension passages is a limited tool for assessing teen health literacy because it was designed for clinical settings and based on reading ability alone. In broader health contexts, a Canadian measurement tool (Wu et al., 2010) has had some success in measuring health literacy in an adolescent population. Other measurement tools include one for media health literacy developed in Israel (Levin-Zamir, Lemish, and Gofin, 2011). There are a number of measurement issues in health literacy that make the evaluation of interventions especially difficult. Most tests have been developed in the US for use in settings within its health care system. Standardized tests are challenging to develop and may be inappropriate in some settings.

There are also more fundamental issues in definitions and testing in general health care settings. In a Canadian study, Begoray and Kwan (2010) found that seniors interpreted key health literacy concepts (e.g., What does it mean to assess health information?) in a variety of ways as meaning everything from looking at the date of the information on a website to considering whether the information agreed with their previous life experience. Complexity in shaping questions will continue to challenge the creation of useful measurement instruments in health literacy.

Knowledge Translation (Theory to Practice)

We need to develop techniques for translating, exchanging, and mobilizing health literacy knowledge into effective lifelong learning practices that take family and community context into account (Banister, Leadbeater, and Marshall, 2011). Some progress in this task has been accomplished by Schecter and Lynch (2011), who suggested that health learning and its presence in adult education needs further theorizing.

The lessons from knowledge translation are useful to investigate lifelong learning in health education in formal school settings as well as other settings. Begoray and Banister (2011) suggested that a promising approach is through community-based, knowledge translation processes based on principles of contextuality (learning suitable to unique environments), collaboration (learning as a social activity), reciprocity (expert and novice learner roles changing according to the learning topics), relationality (building respect between individuals), and reflexivity (becoming more self-aware of personal strengths and challenges). Effective communication and health literacy is paramount to the establishment of these principles.

Increased Emphasis on Mental Health Literacy

With one in five people experiencing mental health challenges and disorders (Canadian Alliance, 2008), mental health literacy needs to be a high priority. The physical, social, and economic costs of stress, anxiety, and mental illness are a major public health issue in developed and developing countries. Mental health literacy promotes a wide range of benefits, including prevention, early recognition, and intervention as well as the reduction of stigma and discrimination that is associated with mental health problems (Canadian Alliance, 2008). However, in order to achieve these benefits, mental health literacy as a concept needs to be more fully investigated and theorized. This will require more definitional work, a comprehensive exploration of its social and developmental aspects, full consideration of the responsibilities of individuals, institutions, and communities as well as basic and applied research in diverse settings to identify effective programs and practices for the broad spectrum of the population (Marshall, 2010). Of particular importance is addressing the stigma that is all too often a deterrent to help seeking behaviours for mental health concerns (Marshall, Davis, and Atherton, 2011; Rickwood et al., 2005).

National mental health education and treatment policies should not be solely concerned with mental disorders but should also recognize and address the broader issues that promote mental health (WHO, 2010). This includes mainstreaming mental health promotion into policies and programs in government, business, education, labour, justice, the environment, housing, and welfare as well as in the health sector itself.

CONCLUSION

The relationship between health literacy and lifelong learning is well established; therefore, we recommend that individuals, communities, health practitioners, and policy makers undertake these practices:

- Provide support and access for people to learn throughout their lives. Education, including adult literacy and health literacy programs, and educational resources must be low cost or free, easily accessible, learner-centred, engaging, and timely. Learning opportunities need to be publicized, easy to locate, and offered by skilled educators and facilitators. Education spending across the life course needs to be a government priority.
- Offer learning as a 'whole person' activity. Learning about health is holistic and more education in one area may well influence learning in other areas. For example, combine learning about health with other learning by improving general literacy; learning another language or new hobbies may lead to new friends and better mental health.
- Design public facilities to foster learning environments for whole communities. Schools for children can become community centres for seniors, clinics (resource centres) for new mothers and infants, exercise space for adults, and even community kitchens. Learning opportunities can feature adolescents helping seniors learn computer skills, seniors helping young children learn how to cook, or adults sharing their arts ability with adolescents.

Questions for Reflection

1) What opportunities for lifelong learning to improve health exist in your community? How might these opportunities be expanded?
2) What do you think are the responsibilities of health care professionals to foster lifelong learning? What responsibility should be borne by individual members of the community?
3) Do you think there is a difference between literacy within the context of health and health literacy? If so, is this distinction important or not?
4) What do you think are opportunities and challenges of integrating health literacy into education practice?
5) Do you consider yourself to be a lifelong learner, both inside and outside the formal educational system? What are your short- and long-term goals for further learning?

ACKNOWLEDGMENTS

We thank Ellahae Kashmiri, Janie Harrison, and Breanna Lawrence, graduate students at the University of Victoria, for their assistance on this chapter.

REFERENCES

Alvermann, D. E., Young, J. P., Green, C., and Wisenbaker, J. M. (1999). Adolescents' perceptions and negotiations of literacy practices in after-school read and talk clubs. *American Educational Research Journal, 36*(2), 221-264. doi:10.3102/00028312036002221.

Banister, E. M., Leadbeater, B. J., and Marshall, E. A. (Eds.). (2011). *Knowledge translation in context: Indigenous, policy, and community settings.* Toronto, Canada: University of Toronto Press.

Begoray, D. L., and Banister, E. M. (2007). Reaching teenagers where they are: Best practices for sexual health education. *Women's Health and Urban Life, 4*(1), 24-40.

Begoray, D. L., and Banister, E. M. (2011). Knowledge translation and adolescent girls' sexual health education in Indigenous communities. In E. M. Banister, E. A. Marshall, and B. J. Leadbeater (Eds.), *Knowledge translation in context: Indigenous, policy and community settings* (pp. 143-160). Toronto, Canada: University of Toronto Press.

Begoray, D. L., Cimon, M., and Wharf-Higgins, J. (2010). *Mediating health: The powerful role of the media.* New York, NY: Nova Science.

Begoray, D. L., and Kwan, B. (2011). A Canadian exploratory study to define a measure of health literacy. *Health Promotion International.* Advance online publication. doi:10.1093/heapro/dar015.

Black, C. (2008). *Working for a healthier tomorrow – Dame Carol Black's review of the health of Britain's working age population.* London, England: The Stationery Office. Available from http://www.dwp.gov.uk/docs/hwwb-working-for-a-healthier-tomorrow.pdf.

Canadian Alliance on Mental Illness and Mental Health. (2008). *National integrated framework for enhancing mental health literacy in Canada: Final report.* Retrieved from http://www.camimh.ca/files/literacy/CAMIMH MHL National Integrated Framework July 2008.pdf.

Canadian Council on Learning. (2009a). *The 2009 composite learning index: Measuring Canada's progress in lifelong learning.* Ottawa, Canada: Author. Retrieved from http://www.nald.ca/library/research/ccl/cli/cli.pdf.

Canadian Council on Learning. (2009b). *2008 survey of Canadian attitudes toward learning: Results for learning throughout the lifespan.* Ottawa, Canada: Author. Retrieved from http://www.nald.ca/library/research/ccl/cli/cli.pdf

Cappon, P. (2006). Connecting the dots on lifelong learning: Canada's new composite learning index. *Policy Options, 27*(9), 78-82.

Chappell, N., and Hollander, M. (2011). An evidence based policy prescription for an aging population. *Healthcare Papers, 11*(1), 8-18. Retrieved from http://www.ncbi.nlm.nih.gov/pubmed/21464622.

Chinn, D. (2011). Critical health literacy: A review and critical analysis. *Social Science and Medicine, 73*, 60-67.

Chisholm, D., and Buchanan, L. (2007). Measuring adolescent functional health literacy: A pilot validation of the test of functional health literacy in adults. *Journal of Adolescent Health, 41*(3), 312-314.

Claxton, G., and Lucas, B. (2009). School as a foundation for lifelong learning: The implications of a lifelong learning perspective for the re-imagining of school-age education. *Inquiry into the Future for Lifelong Learning, 1*, 1-27.

ContinYou. (n.d.). *What is Skilled for Health?* Retrieved from http://www.continyou.org.uk/health_and_well_being/skilled_health/what_skilled_health.

Crick, R. D., Broadfoot, P., and Claxton, G. (2004). Developing an effective lifelong learning inventory: The ELLI project. *Assessment in Education: Principles, Policy and Practice, 11*(3), 247-272. doi:10.1080/0969594042000304582.

Cusack, S. A. (1995). Developing a lifelong learning program: Empowering seniors as leaders in lifelong learning. *Educational Gerontology, 21*(4), 305-320.

Czernochowski, D., Fabiani, M., and Friedman, D. (2008). Use it or lose it? SES mitigates age-related decline in a recency/recognition task. *Neurobiological Aging, 29*(6), 945–958.

Davis, T. C., Wolf, M. S., Bass, P. F., III, Middlebrooks, M., Kennen, E., Baker, D. W.,...Parker, R. M. (2006). Low literacy impairs comprehension of prescription drug warning labels. *Journal of General Internal Medicine, 21*, 847–851. doi:10.1111/j.1525-1497.2006.00529.x.

Field, J. (2005). *Social capital and lifelong learning.* Bristol, England: Policy Press.

Friedman, D. B., and Hoffman-Goetz, L. (2008). Literacy and health literacy as defined in cancer education research: A systematic review. *Health Education Journal, 67*(4), 285-304. doi:10.1177/0017896908097071.

Gonzales, R., Glik, D., Davoudi, M., and Ang, A. (2004). Media literacy and public health. *American Behavioral Scientist, 48*(2), 189-201.

Gray, N. J., Klein, J. D., Noyce, P. R., Sesselberg, T. S., and Cantrill, J. A. (2005). Health information-seeking behaviour in adolescence: The place of the Internet. *Social Science and Medicine, 60*(7), 1467-1478.

Greenberg, M. T., Weissberg, R. P., Utne O'Brien, M., Zins, J. E., Fredricks, L., Resnik, H., and Elias, M. J. (2003). Enhancing school-based prevention and youth development through coordinated social, emotional, and academic learning. *American Psychologist, 58*(6-7), 466-474. doi:10.1037/0003-066X.58.6-7.466.

Griffiths, M. D. (2009). Online computer gaming: Advice for parents and teachers. *Education and Health, 27*(1), 3-6.

Hammond, C. (2004). Impacts of lifelong learning upon emotional resilience, psychological and mental health: Fieldwork evidence. *Oxford Review of Education, 9*(2), 551-567.

Joint Committee on Health Education Terminology. (1991). Report of the 1990 joint committee. *Journal of School Health, 61*, 251-254.

Jorm, A. F., Korten, A. E., Jacomb, P. A., Christensen, H., Rodgers, B., and Pollitt, P. (1997). "Mental health literacy": A survey of the public's ability to recognise mental disorders and their beliefs about the effectiveness of treatment. *Medical Journal of Australia, 166,* 182-186.

Kendall, M. (2005). Lifelong learning really matters for elementary education in the 21st century. *Education and Information Technologies, 10*(3), 289-296.

Kolbe, L. (2005). A framework for school health programs in the 21st century. *Journal of School Health, 75*(6), 226-228.

Levin-Zamir, D., Lemish, D., and Gofin, R. (2011). Media health literacy (MHL): Development and measurement of the concept among adolescents. *Health Education Research, 26*(2), 323-335.

Li, J., Mattes, E., Stanley, F., McMurray, A., and Hertzman, C. (2009). Social determinants of child health and well being. *Health Sociology Review, 18,* 3–11.

Longworth, N., and Davies, W. K. (1996). *Lifelong learning.* London, England: Kogan Page.

Manganello, J. (2008). Health literacy and adolescents: A framework and agenda for future research. *Health Education Research, 23,* 840-847.

Marshall, E. A. (2010, February). *Mental health literacy across the lifespan.* Paper presented at the Health Literacy: Making the Most of Health Conference, London, England.

Marshall, E. A., Davis, M., and Atherton, M. A. (2011). *Caring minds: Addressing mental health stigma among adolescents.* Manuscript submitted for publication.

Mayhew, M., Wolniak, G., and Pascarella, E. (2008). How educational practices affect the development of life-long learning orientations in traditionally-aged undergraduate students. *Research in Higher Education, 49,* 337-356.

Mitchell, B., and Begoray, D. L. (2010). Electronic personal health records that promote self-management in chronic illness. *OJIN: The Online Journal of Issues in Nursing, 15*(3). doi:10.3912/OJIN.Vol15No03PPT01.

Natharius, D. (2004). The more we know, the more we see: The role of visuality in media literacy. *American Behavioral Scientist, 48*(2), 238-247.

New London Group. (1996). A pedagogy of multiliteracies: Designing social futures. *Harvard Educational Review, 66*(1), 60-92.

Nutbeam, D. (2000). Health literacy as a public health goal: A challenge for contemporary health education and communication strategies into the 21st century. *Health Promotion International, 15*(3), 259-267.

Nutbeam, D. (2008). The evolving concept of health literacy. *Social Science and Medicine, 67*(12), 2072-2078.

Organisation for Economic Co-operation and Development and Statistics Canada. (1995). *Literacy, economy and society: Results of the first international adult literacy survey.* Paris, France and Ottawa, Canada: Authors.

Peattie, S. (2007). The internet as a medium for communicating with teenagers. *Social Marketing Quarterly, XIII*(2), 21-46.

Perrin, B. (1998). *How does literacy affect the health of Canadians? A profile paper.* Ottawa, Canada: Health Promotion and Programs Branch, Health Canada. Retrieved from http://www.nald.ca/library/research/howdoes/howdoes.pdf.

Porter, R., and Fraser, A. (2006). *Royal College of General Practitioners Curriculum statement 10.2: Men's health.* London, England: Royal College of General Practitioners. Available from http://www.rcgp.org.uk/pdf/educ_curr10.2%20Mens%20health%20Feb%2006.pdf.

Prensky, M. (2001). *Digital natives, digital immigrants.* Retrieved from http://www.marcprensky.com/writing/.

Rayner, G., and Lang, T. (2011). Is nudge an effective public health strategy to tackle obesity? No. *British Medical Journal, 342.* doi:10.1136/bmj.d2177.

Reiss, G., Gibson, W., and Walker, L. (2005). Health care transition: Youth family, and provider perspectives. *Paediatrics, 115*(1), 112-120.

Rickwood, D., Dean, F. P., Wilson, C. J., and Ciarrochi, J. (2005). Young people's help-seeking for mental health problems. *Advances in Mental Health 4*(S3), S218-251.

Rideout, V., Roberts, D. F., and Foehr, U. G. (2005). *Generation M: Media in the lives of 8-18 year olds.* Menlo Park, CA: Kaiser Family Foundation.

Ronson, B., and Rootman, I. (2009). Literacy: One of the most important determinants of health. In D. Raphael (Ed.), *Social determinants of health: Canadian perspectives* (2nd ed., pp. 170-185). Toronto, Canada: Canadian Scholars' Press.

Rootman, I., and Edwards, P. (2004). The best laid schemes of mice and men. ParticipACTION's legacy and the future of physical activity promotion in Canada. *Canadian Journal of Public Health, 95*(S2), S37-42.

Rootman, I., and Gordon-El-Bihbety, D. (2008). *A vision for a health literate Canada: Report of the expert panel on health literacy.* Ottawa, Canada: Canadian Public Health Association.

Schecter, S. R., and Lynch, J. (2011). Health learning and adult education: In search of a theory of practice. *Adult Education Quarterly, 61*, 207-224. doi:10.1177/0741713610380438.

Simpson, K., and Freeman, R. (2004). Critical health promotion and education: A new research challenge. *Health Education Research, 19*(3), 340-348.

Skilled for Health. (n.d.). *Making the case*. Retrieved from http://rwp.qia.oxi.net/embeddedlearning/skilled_health/index.cfm.

Statistics Canada. (2007). *Study: Using the internet for education purposes*. Ottawa, Canada: Author. Retrieved from http://www.statcan.ca/Daily/ English/071030/d071030b.htm.

Tavistock Institute and Shared Intelligence. (2009). *Evaluation of the second phase of the Skilled for Health Programme: Final evaluation report*. London, England: Authors.

Tones, K. (2002). Health literacy: New wine in old bottles? *Health Education Research, 17*(3), 287-290.

Tylee, A., Haller, D. M., Graham, T., Churchill, R., and Sanci, L. A. (2007). Youth-friendly primary care services: How are we doing and what more needs to be done? *The Lancet, 369*(9572), 1565-1573.

United Kingdom Department of Business, Innovation and Skills. (2010). *Skills for sustainable growth: Executive summary*. London, England: Author. Retrieved from http://www.bis.gov.uk/assets/biscore/further-education-skills/docs/s/10-1273-skills-for-sustainable-growth-strategy-summary.pdf.

von Wagner, C., Steptoe, A., Wolf, M., and Wardle, J. (2009). Health literacy and health actions: A review and framework from health psychology. *Health Education and Behavior, 36*(5), 860-877.

Vygotsky, L. (1978). *Mind in society: The development of higher psychological processes*. Cambridge, MA: Harvard University Press.

Washington State Department of Health. (2011). *Adolescent health transition project website*. Retrieved from http://depts.washington.edu/healthtr/.

Weiss, B. D., Blanchard, J. S., McGee, D. L., Hart, G., Warren, B., Burgoon, M., and Smith, K. J. (1994). Illiteracy among Medicaid recipients and its relationship to health care costs. *Journal of Health Care for the Poor and Underserved, 5*(2), 99-111.

Wharf-Higgins, J., Begoray, D. L., and MacDonald, M. (2009). A social ecological conceptual framework for understanding adolescent health literacy in the health education classroom. *American Journal of Community Psychology, 16*(4), 350-362. doi:10.1007/s10464-009-9270-8.

Wister, A.V., Malloy-Weir, L. J., Rootman, I., and Desjardins, R. (2010). Lifelong educational practices and resources in enabling health literacy among older adults. *Journal of Aging and Health, 22*(6), 827-854.

Wolf, M. S., Wilson, E. A., Rapp, D. N., Waite, K. R., Bocchini, M. V., Davis, T. C., and Rudd, R. E. (2009). Literacy and learning in health care. *Paediatrics, 124*(3), 275-281.

World Health Organization. (1948). *Preamble to the constitution of the World Health Organization.* Geneva, Switzerland: Author. Retrieved from http://apps.who.int/gb/bd/PDF/BD47/EN/constitution-en.pdf.

World Health Organization. (1998). *Health promotion glossary.* Geneva, Switzerland: Author.

World Health Organization. (2010, September). *Mental health: Strengthening our response.* (Fact Sheet No. 220). Geneva, Switzerland: Author. Retrieved from http://www.who.int/mediacentre/factsheets/fs220/en/.

Wu, A. D., Begoray, D. L., MacDonald, M., Wharf-Higgins, J., Frankish, J., Kwan, B., … Rootman, I. (2010). Developing and evaluating a relevant and feasible instrument for measuring health literacy of Canadian high school students. *Health Promotion International.* Advance online publication. doi:10.1093/heapro/daq032.

In: Health Literacy in Context   ISBN: 978-1-61942-921-5
Eds.: D.Begoray, D.Gillis, G.Rowlands © 2012 Nova Science Publishers, Inc.

Chapter 6

HEALTH LITERACY, CULTURE, AND COMMUNITY

Diane Levin-Zamir[*] and Jane Wills

ABSTRACT

This chapter explores the relationship between health literacy, culture and community. The notion of community with regard to health literacy focuses on groups within the population that identify themselves as having common culture, values, and/or needs and share a commitment to meeting them. The health literacy challenges of specific groups within communities (e.g., older adults, migrants, immigrants, and cultures in transition from traditional to western societies) are reviewed and discussed. The implications of virtual communities on health literacy are raised. Among these groups, navigating and making decisions related to the health system are emphasized. Examples of health literacy interventions among specific cultures in communities through literature review and case studies from the United Kingdom and Israel are presented. Gaps in present research are noted, particularly with regard to effectiveness of interventions; directions for future research and participatory action in the community are proposed.

[*] Corresponding author: E-mail: diamos@zahav.net.il.

INTRODUCTION

There are many definitions of health literacy (see Chapter 2). In this chapter, we adopt the World Health Organization (WHO) definition because it is most consistent with the health promotion and community focus of the chapter:

> represent(ing) the cognitive and social skills which determine the motivation and ability of individuals to gain access to, understand and use information in ways which promote and maintain good health. Health literacy means more than being able to read pamphlets and successfully make appointments. By improving people's access to health information and their capacity to use it effectively health literacy is critical to empowerment. (WHO, 1998, p. 10)

Central to this definition is the concept of empowerment and individuals' ability to take control of their health. The concept of health literacy has generated both interest and debate in defining the term while seeking to understand whether and how health literacy impacts health outcomes and health inequalities (see Chapter 2). This has created considerable interest in working with communities experiencing these poor health outcomes to improve their functional literacy and thereby their ability to use health information and navigate health care systems. We focus on understanding the communities of interest in relation to the development of health literacy in the broader sense of the concept as defined by WHO.

Functional literacy is associated with greater educational achievement, sustainable livelihoods, and better health in both developed and developing countries. Low health literacy as functionally measured is associated with worse health outcomes (Kutner, Greenberg, Jin, and Paulsen, 2006). Both literacy and health literacy are more likely to be lacking in specific population groups (e.g., migrants and refugees, older people, minority ethnic groups, lower socioeconomic groups). Thus, health literacy is understood as a risk or attribute whose absence may severely affect health outcomes; on the other hand, it may be developed or acquired as an outcome of specific interventions.

Critical and interactive health literacy are different categories of health literacy (Nutbeam, 2000, 2008) that link it with education and empowerment, deviating from a more clinical perspective, characterizing it as an issue that patients and health professionals need to address (Pleasant and Kuruvilla, 2008). As such, these categories refer to the skills and capabilities that promote community action for health and focus on the higher-level cognitive and social skills required to analyse and use information to understand the social, economic, and environmental determinants of health and then to exert greater control over life events and situations through individual and collective action (Chinn, 2011). Key to discussions of health literacy and communities is whether health-literate communities are those that understand the conditions influencing their health and have the knowledge and skills to change them—perhaps similar to what is defined by Freedman et al. (2009) as public health literacy.

Kickbush (2001) noted that the concept of critical health literacy derives from community development approaches, centred on a Freircian model of critical consciousness (Freire, 1970) and based on an education of questioning, including questions regarding the learners' social conditions. Thus, teaching words becomes a means to teaching about the world rather than an end in itself. In this conceptualisation, health literacy is not dependent on basic reading and writing skills as has been shown in countries with low levels of literacy, such as China and Bangladesh (Jahan, 2000; Wang, 2000) but has social action as the centre of the learning. Papen (2009) suggested that those who might be regarded as lacking literacy skills can still mobilize social resources and social capital to make sense of health information.

HEALTH LITERACY AND COMMUNITIES

There is no universal definition of the term *community*. Most commonly cited factors considered in conceptualizing community are geography, culture, and social stratification, which are linked to the subjective feeling of belonging or identity. In this chapter, a combination of definitions is adopted. First, WHO (1998) defined communities as: "A specific group of people, often living in a defined geographic area, who share a common culture, values and norms .... They exhibit some awareness of their identity as a group and share common needs and a commitment to meeting them" (p. 5). Second, the National Institute for Health and Clinical Excellence (2007) defined community as "social or family groups linked by networks, geographical location or another common factor" (p. 38). Furthermore, the community is characterized as a *setting*, first mentioned in the Lalonde Paper (1974) on the health of Canadians and as indicated in the *Ottawa Charter for Health Promotion*: "health is created and lived by people within the settings of their everyday life; where they learn, work, play and love" (WHO, 1986, p. 3).

People in particular settings (e.g., schools or health services) may be seen as comprising a community. For example, patients with specific conditions can be considered a community, sharing common characteristics in expert patients' programmes that support patients in exercising greater levels of expertise in managing long-term conditions (National Primary Care and Research Development Centre, 2006).

We can see different interpretations of community and different rationales for directing specific policy or practice to a particular community. An ethical rationale argues that targeting the most vulnerable and marginalized is needed to supplement a universal service if the needs of all population groups are to be met equally. An economic rationale argues that it is more cost-effective to provide resources to meet needs effectively rather than spend resources later to address the multiple social effects (e.g., acute and chronic ill health) resulting from a failure to meet needs. A scientific rationale rests on a notion of risk. Epidemiological evidence identifies population groups on the basis of their behavioural risk factors, environmental risk conditions, their health outcomes (i.e., ill health or premature death), or ease of access to care and services (Naidoo and Wills, 2010).

In the late twentieth century, many developed countries shared a political philosophy that the community was the site where needs are both defined and met and that some population groups such as migrants or older people are marginalized, harder to reach, or excluded from mainstream services. For example, in the United Kingdom (UK), the concept of social inclusion/exclusion gained currency as a way of focusing on populations that do not make use of opportunities to participate in society. Under the coalition government created in 2010, the concept of community acquired a different meaning. Political efforts attempted to build the 'Big Society' in which power will be transferred from the state to people, individuals, neighbourhoods, or communities using lay people in the delivery of care—both as volunteers and in non-professional paid roles (Cabinet Office, 2010).

In the US, the Asset-Based Community Development (ABCD) Institute (http://www.abcdinstitute.org) focuses on local assets as the building blocks of sustainable community development. Building on the skills of local residents, the power of local associations, and the supportive functions of local institutions, ABCD draws upon existing community strengths to build stronger, more sustainable communities. Such communities may then be said to have developed critical health literacy in understanding the social determinants of their health (e.g., transport, isolation, housing) and taking action to tackle them.

When the promotion of health literacy with communities is explored, there is a key distinction between the promotion of functional literacy with groups/communities and community development that seeks to develop critical health literacy. Interventions to promote the health literacy of communities and their ability to use information may be based in a community or setting but are quite individualist; the goal is for the user of health care or health information to become autonomous and responsible. For the practitioner, the focus is on changing communication practices to be more appropriate whether by recognizing culturally and linguistically diverse communities and then providing translated materials, developing cultural competency or through advocates and care navigators. The assumption is that communities or groups with poor health outcomes are not understanding and/or applying health-related information to adopt healthy lifestyles and self-care.

An alternative view of health literacy and communities references what Chinn (2011) called the "collectivist-minded, socially active citizen who prioritizes the common good and public health goals" (p. 65) or critical health literacy. Porr, Drummond, and Richter (2006) described a project with low-income mothers in Australia in which the health care professional facilitates exploration of topics or problems (e.g., inadequate financial support, lack of affordable housing, transportation concerns); the underlying commonality is that they have affected the lives of the mothers, thus leaving them powerless. The search for the sources of powerlessness goes beyond the individual to the surrounding economic, social, and political forces. The young women in the study were encouraged to exchange ideas and identify issues during group dialogue, which would progress to action plans and campaigns for change.

HEALTH LITERACY AND CULTURE

In this chapter, culture is defined as "the learned and shared behavior of a community of interacting human beings" (Useem, Useem, and Donoghue, 1963, p. 169) and "the integrated system learned behaviour patterns which are characteristic of the members of a society" (Hoebel and Frost, 1976, p. 6). The United States (US) Department of Health and Human Services (HHS) Office of Minority Health (2000b) defined culture as integrated patterns of human behaviour that include the language, thoughts, communications, actions, customs, beliefs, values, and institutions of racial, ethnic, religious, or social groups. Culture in the context of health and health behaviour relates to the shared values, beliefs, and practices "to find meaningful, structured modes of social interactions interpersonally and institutionally to support the well-being of its members." (Kagawa-Singer, 2011, p. S90). Whilst health literacy is dependent upon many factors (e.g., education, past experience with the health system, age, gender), it is also influenced by cultural background (HHS, 2000; Nielsen-Bohlman, Panzer, and Kindig, 2004). Thus, health systems in general, and those in the community in particular, must become culturally competent and responsive to health literacy needs. Cultural competence in health care describes the ability of systems to provide care to patients with diverse values, beliefs and behaviours, including tailoring delivery to meet patients' social, cultural, and linguistic needs (Betancourt, Green, and Carrillo, 2002). Cultural competence in the context of health literacy includes four aspects: (a) cultural awareness or sensitivity to values, beliefs, and lifestyles that stem from one's culture; (b) cultural knowledge, including educational foundation concerning worldviews of various cultures; (c) cultural skill or the ability to collect (verbal and physical) relevant cultural data regarding clients' health histories and presenting problems; and (d) cultural encounter or crosscultural interactions with clients from culturally diverse backgrounds (US Institute of Medicine [IOM], 2002).

The importance of understanding the association between cultural competency, community empowerment, and health literacy is based on three pillars. First, the concepts together form a basis for improving measurable health indicators. Second, the empowerment–cultural competence–health literacy connection has significance regarding the use of public resources for health care. The IOM (Nielsen-Bohlman, et al., 2004) estimated that the health care cost of low health literacy, due in part to cultural disparities, is approximately $50–73 billion a year, which is the equivalent to approximately €37–50 billion or £30–44 billion. These costs stem from increased need for repeated examinations, treatments, and hospitalizations due to mistakes in communication and misunderstandings, etc. Third, a heavy price is paid at the individual level due to damaged self-esteem caused by frequently formidable encounters with the health care system. The lack of interpersonal communication avenues, culturally adapted to the individual, are frequently a source of embarrassment and shame—so much so that within certain cultural systems, individuals are prohibited from expressing their needs to health care providers or to other individuals in their immediate surroundings (American Medical Association [AMA] Ad Hoc Committee on Health Literacy, 1999; Parihk, Parker, Nurss, Baker, and Williams, 1996).

The relationship between the health systems and cultural systems can be understood using Foster's (1978) model of universal health systems. This model maintains that every culture has a health system consisting of four components: the cause of disease, symptoms, diagnosis, and treatment/cure. Each culture has a designated individual whose function is to treat exceptional health situations. Western medical systems usually function in a linear, chronological paradigm. Furthermore, western medicine has embraced the notion of asymptomatic health situations. Traditional medical systems are known to embrace a more complex model, with the sociocultural identity at the centre of the system and the cause, symptom, diagnosis, and treatment branching out from this central identity, not necessarily in the said chronological sequence (Levin, 1980). When western and traditional health systems meet—as in the case with migrants, immigrants, Aboriginal Peoples, and cultures in transition, research has shown that the component of the traditional health system most flexible to change is the notion of treatment. Least likely to change is the perception of cause of disease, which is highly associated with sociocultural identity.

Increasingly, health care professionals have to provide care and education to diverse patient populations who have cultural, linguistic, and health literacy barriers (Nova Scotia Department of Health, 2010). Strategies recommended in order to enhance health literacy through culturally appropriate health systems include training staff to create a shame-free environment, enhancing assessment techniques, improving culturally responsive interpersonal communication skills, creating and using patient-friendly written materials and signage, and developing and implementing sustainable, effective interventions (AMA, 1999).

HEALTH LITERACY AND COMMUNITIES: REVIEW OF RESEARCH

A rapid review of published research on health literacy and communities reveals various conceptualizations of the concept of community categorized by life course (e.g., older or younger people), cultural and linguistic communities, and cyber or virtual communities. Additionally, health literacy research has studied settings (e.g., schools), populations with low functional literacy (e.g., offenders), and people with specific conditions (e.g., diabetes). The nature of the research is skewed toward cross-sectional studies that measure the prevalence of levels of health literacy and their determinants and the association with health outcomes. Fewer studies examine health literacy and community-based interventions (Canadian Public Health Association, 2006; King, 2007). While the community can be a basis for intervention and advocacy for reducing health disparities in communities and for promoting critical health literacy, most studies that examined the association between health literacy and health focused on functional health literacy, with little or no examination of critical or interactive health literacy (Nutbeam, 2000).

Health Literacy and Older Adults in Community Settings

The health literacy of older adults has been researched over the past decade. They have more chronic illnesses, use more health care services than other segments of the population, and face unique issues related to physical and cognitive functioning—all making it difficult to find and use appropriate health information (HHS, 2000a). Literacy surveys reveal that people aged 65 and older have the smallest proportion of proficient health literacy skills (Kutner et al., 2006). A recent review of health literacy among older adults (Zamora and Clingerman, 2011) found that advancing age results in a significant increase in prevalence of inadequate health literacy. Older people living independently in community settings are more likely than the rest of the adult population to be challenged with numerous cognitive processes involved in navigating health care systems: retrieving prescriptions and referrals, selecting providers from a list of names and addresses, calculating when to take multiple medications, and interpreting medical terminology (Kintsch, 1998). Studies show the association between low functional health literacy among the elderly and adverse health outcomes, such as higher hospitalization rates, an inability to manage chronic diseases, and increased mortality (Baker et al., 2007; Gazmararian, Williams, Peel, and Baker, 2003; Sudore et al., 2006). Gazmararian et al. (2003) studied adults receiving Medicare and living in the community with chronic diseases; they found that health literacy level proved to be an independent predictor of patients' knowledge of their chronic illness, even after controlling for age, disease duration, and prior attendance at a disease-specific education class.

Conclusions from these studies highlight the need for enabling better communication in health care contexts, whether routine or unexpected, and for enhancing the ability of older adults to follow treatment instructions and to find, understand, and evaluate health information. Further research is needed to develop evidence-based, culturally congruent interventions to improve health literacy among older adults.

Health Literacy and Culturally and Linguistically Diverse Communities

The 2003 National Assessment of Adult Literacy in the US (Kutner et al., 2006) measured health literacy in several culturally diverse populations. The health literacy scores for Black, Hispanic, and American Indian/Alaskan Native populations were lower than White and Asian adults. These health literacy disparities contribute to ethnic and racial disparities and vice versa. Communicating effectively with immigrant and migrant populations is a complex matter (Kreps and Sparks, 2008). The significant language and health literacy difficulties faced by immigrant populations are frequently exacerbated by cultural barriers and economic challenges to accessing health services. In addition, people's responses to illness are culturally determined and may be expressed differently in response to illness, including how they express and articulate fear, pain, and anxiety and define *sick roles*. The concept of health as well as illness varies widely across cultural groups.

Health literacy is a critical determinant of a person's ability to navigate the health care system, fill out forms, share information and personal history, locate service providers, and engage in chronic disease management. Numerous studies explore how people with specific conditions from new immigrant groups are informed and educated about their condition (e.g., Barrera-Anderson, Olives, Larsen, and Periera, 2007; Thomson and Hoffman-Goetz, 2011). Zanchetta and Poureslami (2006) described some of the problems faced by new arrivals in Canada: health professionals who cannot communicate effectively, educational resources and approaches that only partially reach people from cultural minorities, and eHealth information that does little for those with language and literacy limitations. A systematic review by Poureslami, Rootman, Balka, Devarakonda, Hatch, and Fitzgerald (2007) found studies addressed similar themes in relation to asthma management in Canada including patient education, approaches to language limitation and cultural barriers, studies of health care system bias (in terms of culturally competent care), and attempts to facilitate participatory decision making by both provider and patient.

There is limited evidence, however, on effective interventions with culturally and linguistically diverse communities. Simich (2009) found few good practice examples that included clear writing and oral communication (between patients and health care professionals), training for health professionals targeting low-literate groups, and visual tools (e.g., video and other non-written means of communication). Simich described some promising health promotion and community-based interventions usually performed by a health educator who is linguistically competent and culturally acceptable to the community involved.

Health Literacy and Virtual Communities

The concept of communities and settings has not only a geographical or organizational form but also a virtual one, particularly among adolescents. The need for understanding more about the role media plays in health literacy among adolescents has been demonstrated (Begoray, Wharf-Higgins, and MacDonald, 2009). The widespread use of the Internet as a source of information and social network is increasingly being documented. The Pew Internet project in the US examined the social life of the Internet and its impact on health (Fox, 2011). Through listserve, discussion groups, and forums, it serves as a medium whereby communities of patients sharing the same chronic condition can share observations with one another. A systematic review (Eysenbach, Powell, Englesakin, Rizo, and Stern, 2004) of health and the new media found a lack of measurable evidence from controlled studies in sharp contrast to the increasing body of anecdotal and descriptive information on self-help processes in virtual communities. Given the abundance of unmoderated peer-to-peer groups on the Internet, Eysenbach et al. (2004) concluded that research is required to evaluate under which conditions and for whom electronic support groups are effective, including maximizing social support.

Recently, the concept and measurement instruments of Media Health Literacy (MHL) were developed and tested among adolescents. MHL is defined as "the ability to identify health-related content (explicit and/or implicit) in the media; recognize its influence on health behavior...; [to] critically analyze the content ... and to express intention to respond through action" (Levin-Zamir, Lemish, and Gofin, 2011, p. 325). The use of this new concept and measurement tool is the basis for interventions underway that are focused on improving MHL among adolescents in the community.

HEALTH LITERACY, CULTURE, AND COMMUNITY — CASE STUDIES

Following this discussion of health literacy, culture, and community, it can be concluded that most of the literature has centered on either theoretical discourse or reports of findings from cross-sectional surveys. The following examples describe action-based interventions building on the important ties between the health literacy, culture, and community. These examples describe an analysis from the literature of approaches to promote health literacy with one ethnic community in the UK and the field experience from two culturally adapted community interventions based on health literacy needs in Israel.

Gypsy, Roma, and Travellers in the UK

The UK Context

Western societies frequently espouse policies of tolerance in respect of diversity within society. Since the 1950s, Britain has experienced the development of substantial visible-minority communities including people from present and former Commonwealth countries and more recently from Eastern European countries as part of migration within the European Union. Minority languages, religions, and cultural practices have been encouraged; and rights and freedoms were enshrined in legislation covering race relations and public order. Health services and social care are universal services free at the point of delivery in the UK, and access to other services such as education, employment, and housing is expected to be open to all without discrimination. Respect for cultural particularity and diversity has, however, recently been criticised for potentially undermining social and national cohesion; and multiculturalism is being reframed to establish commonality and cohesion through shared national values—what Prime Minister David Cameron (2011) has called "state multiculturalism" (para. 8).

Case Study

Earlier in this chapter we described some of the challenges in defining the concept of community. Gypsy, Roma, and Travellers is a collective term used to describe a variety of cultural and ethnic groups whose language, history, and nomadic way of life may differ. But crucially, they self-identify as Gypsy, Roma, and Traveller—a term that is generally acceptable to these groups.

The following case study highlights the inequalities faced by approximately half a million people in Gypsy, Roma, and Traveller communities who were recognised as a distinct ethnic group in 1989. It illustrates the extent to which many of their experiences remain invisible and ignored despite this agenda of respect for diversity and universal access to services. Much of the focus on the inequalities experienced by this population group relates to their insecure accommodation and unauthorised encampments and developments, but they also experience a lack of access to provisions and services taken for granted by the mainstream population. Since about 2000, governments have been concerned with groups of people who are cut off or socially excluded from mainstream society, whose needs are complex, and who are particularly difficult to reach. The Labour government established a social inclusion institute, later to become a social exclusion task force that has been absorbed into the coalition government's Office for Civil Society. Gypsies, Roma, and Travellers are frequently excluded from the concept of exclusion itself, from policies to address it, and from ethnic monitoring and equity audits that attempt to monitor service use and reduce inequalities (Cemlyn, Greenfields, Burnett, Matthews, and Whitwell, 2009).

Reported health problems of Gypsy, Roma, and Travellers are two to five times more prevalent in this community than amongst UK comparator populations in relation to self-reported anxiety, respiratory problems including asthma and bronchitis, and chest pain (Cemlyn et al., 2009). The excess prevalence of miscarriages, stillbirths, neonatal deaths, and premature death of older offspring is also conspicuous (Parry et al., 2004).

Much of the information and research around the health of Gypsy, Roma, and Travellers is rooted in a biomedical rather than social model of health, which has led to the cause of these challenging public health problems to be attributed to their behaviour—either their lack of education and illiteracy or the pathologisation of their lifestyle and culture. Poor literacy levels and a consequent lack of knowledge of health systems are cited in numerous needs assessments as barriers to accessing health services and information (Cemlyn et al., 2009). Complex and variable letter-and-form based appointment systems may well contribute to reluctance to engage with health services because of a sense of shame or humiliation related to the poor literacy skills that is common to this population (Van Cleemput, Thomas, Parry, Peters, and Cooper, 2007). Several studies reported that Gypsy, Roma, and Travellers have difficulty in understanding advice given by health professionals, and the use of jargon is a barrier to accessing effective health care (Cemlyn et al., 2009). Consequent frustration by health care professionals may be perceived by Gypsy, Roma, and Travellers as unwarranted aggression or rudeness. Van Cleemput (2008) reported that: "Shame and attempts to ward off shame are central features of relationships and encounters with health staff, as personal reactions to these experiences can produce mutual mistrust and poor relations between staff and the Gypsy and Traveller patients." (as cited in Cemlyn et al., 2009, p. 53).

Most approaches to working with Gypsy, Roma, and Traveller communities adopt what could be referred to as a deficit-based approach in which illiteracy is seen as a barrier to health that can be remedied by education programmes. Primary care organizations have health service information routinely translated into ethnic minority languages and also produce information in audio form (tape/video/CD). Some health professionals act as brokers into health services (e.g., health visitors, community midwives, etc.) but usually on an ad hoc basis (Cemlyn et al., 2009).

Reviews of interventions (e.g., Cemlyn et al., 2009) concluded that community-based advocacy is more likely to be effective than health education, whether this is through resources and materials or one-to-one advice. A project in Sussex (Sussex Traveller Women's Health Project, n.d.) utilised a method of community development in which a Gypsy Traveller outreach worker visited, sited, and housed Travellers and then set up support and education groups in different localities based on Traveller women's self-identified health needs. The women then acted as peer educators and advocates for others. The education and advocacy work of the women evolved to becoming a link between statutory health agencies and the Travelling community, helping to reduce the real or perceived mistrust that is commonly held by both practitioners and Travelling community members (Parry et al., 2004; Van Cleemput, 2008).

This example typifies the Freireian approaches to adult education described previously in which a dialogue between learner and educator leads to critical consciousness-raising such that adult learners become aware of the causes of their oppression that in turn becomes a basis for action (Freire, 1970). Smart, Titterton, and Clark (2003) suggested that such an approach is recommended with Gypsy, Roma, and Traveller communities instead of literacy schemes or the use of health advocates; it is asset rather than deficit based, challenging exclusion and discrimination, and celebrating cultures and traditions.

The Gypsy, Roma, and Traveller communities illustrate different perspectives in promoting health literacy. The communities experience disproportionate health problems, frequently attributed to underutilisation of services that is, in turn, attributed to their limited functional literacy. The conventional response has been to develop literacy and numeracy skills to encourage the Gypsy, Roma, and Travellers to better utilise health promotion and screening services. Yet these communities are often illustrative of high levels of critical health literacy in their ability to tackle some of the social determinants of their health, such as housing settlement and environmental waste.

The Israeli Context

For over 60 years, Israel has been the focus of migration of multitudes of people from many countries who bring with them an understanding of health and disease with different experiences related to health care. The multicultural mosaic of Israeli society warrants the development of culturally appropriate intervention strategies for enhancing empowerment based on health literacy. The notion of cultural competence and health literacy is extremely relevant in the Israeli context, particularly as it relates to immigrant (e.g., Russian, Ethiopian), migrant (e.g., foreign workers from the Philippines and Eastern Europe), and cultures in transition (e.g., Haredi or Arabic cultures).

Two specific interventions are described as well as their results; the first was implemented among the Ethiopian immigrant population and the second among the older Arab population. All residents in Israel, including immigrants, are entitled to universal health care coverage and choose one of four health service organizations for their health care. The interventions described were initiated by Clalit Health Services, Israel's largest health service organization and the second largest non-governmental health service organization in the world. The organization has over 1,350 community care clinics, 14 hospitals, over 400 pharmacies, and hundreds of additional health service facilities. Clalit provides comprehensive health care to most (54%) of Israel's population, including 80% of Israel's elderly population, 75% of the Arab community, 83% of the Ethiopian community, and a significantly higher rate of the population with low socioeconomic status as compared to the other health care organizations in Israel. The organizational structure facilitates cooperation between primary health community clinics and hospitals as well as collaboration with non-governmental organizations and community services.

Community Case Study 1: Refuah Shlema — Cultural Liaisons in the Community

Since the first major wave of Ethiopian immigrants to Israel in the 1980s and continuing through the 1990s, voices from the Ethiopian community expressed a dire need for culturally appropriate communication, better access to health information, more understanding of health care providers, and wider access to health resources. Ethiopian immigrants experienced significant adjustment challenges regarding use of health services due to cultural disparities (Epstein, 2006); examples included cross-cultural communication problems and discrepancies in the cultural perspectives and habits regarding health in general and, more specifically, the primary care system in the community (Levin-Zamir, Lipsky, Goldberg, and Melamud, 1993).

In 1997, Clalit developed the *Refuah Shlema* programme with a variety of partners and ultimately with the Ministry of Health (Levin-Zamir, Keret et al., 2011).The objective of the programme is to promote the health of the Ethiopian community through improved communication between primary care workers (i.e., physicians, nurses, pharmacists, administrative staff) and immigrants based on health literacy. It includes three interventions:

- Employing Ethiopian health liaisons as cultural mediators in primary care community clinics throughout Israel.
- In-service training of clinic staff to improve cultural competence and bridge cross-cultural gaps.
- Community-wide health education activities for Ethiopian immigrants tailored to the needs of each community.

Evidence of the effectiveness of Refuah Shlema is based on data from a variety of sources gathered using qualitative and quantitative methods. Satisfaction, perceived access to care, improved communication and treatment of patients as perceived by the health care provider funders/health system policy makers, and costs to the community health system, including the use of medical services by the community, were all analyzed early on (Nirel, Rosen, and Ismail, 2000). Research tools were culturally adapted to the Ethiopian community promote validity and cultural sensitivity. The results of the intervention clinics were compared to those of the clinics that had not yet begun the programme.

Findings from 666 in-depth interviews in Amaharic with Ethiopian immigrants from a range of age groups and number of years in Israel as well aswith clinic staff showed that the Ethiopian cultural mediators contributed greatly to building trust and confidence in efficacy of treatments and in accepting health recommendations. Open-ended questionnaires, developed using a participatory approach, facilitated an understanding of the needs of community clinic staff before and after the in-service training. Group discussions with the staff elicited information needed to understand the contribution of the capacity-building component and to determine what was lacking in support of their work with the immigrants.

Data on per capita expenditures before and several years after the launch of the programme were analyzed. An index for costs for prescription medication, referral to and use of tertiary medical services, and hospitalization was developed. Community health status was measured through national quality health indicators for the communities participating in the Refuah Shlema programme. Without the programme, indicators lower than the national average were expected due to the known influence of cultural adjustment as a social determinant of health.

The findings showed that the Refuah Shlema clinics had average or above average rates of health quality indicators when compared to the national or district standards. The programme was positively associated with improved ability to navigate the health system, without increasing public or individual expenditure on services. Data showed that unnecessary medical tests were performed in clinics where the programme was not implemented. It not only met the needs of the immigrants living in the community but was also instrumental in attracting new families to the community due to improved access to the western health system, otherwise highly disenfranchising.

The evaluation of the capacity-building efforts showed heightened cultural sensitivity among participating primary care staff. The staff members were interested in improving cultural competence to provide better services to the community. Meetings regularly held for capacity building and support of the national group of cultural liaisons have been sustained for nearly 15 years. The programme is currently implemented in 25 community clinics serving over 30% of the Ethiopian community in Israel. The scope is a result of advocacy among policy makers and stakeholders. An annual budget for this programme from at least two major public sources (i.e., Clalit Health Services and the Israel Ministry of Health) is allocated each year. This is the longest community intervention programme sustained in Israel, rooted in cultural competency and health literacy (Levin-Zamir, 2011).

Community Case Study 2: Community Intervention for Diabetes Control among the Adult Arab Population

Cultural competency principles were applied to health literacy in a national initiative for improving diabetes control among the Arab population in Israel. Type 2 diabetes mellitus is becoming more prevalent among cultures in transition from traditional to western lifestyles (Hossain, Kawar, and El Nahas, 2007). The prevalence of Type 2 diabetes in Israel is 5.9% in adults, compared to the prevalence of diabetes in non-Hispanic white populations in the western world, which is 8%. The prevalence of diabetes in the Israeli Arab population is three times higher than the Jewish population, attributed to change in lifestyles including lack of physical activity and unhealthy eating habits. Complications of diabetes are attributed to the high rate of cigarette smoking among Arab males. A national programme for diabetes control has been conducted for 12 years within which a special initiative for the Arab population was planned, implemented, and evaluated (Goldracht et al., 2011).

Goals

The goals of the national intervention programme were to:

- increase awareness in the Arab community regarding diabetes, the importance of treatment, and reduce the existing stigma regarding chronic disease;
- develop and apply a lifestyle change programme, culturally tailored to the Arab community, focusing on nutrition, physical activity, smoking cessation, and foot care.

The national intervention programme initiated by the Clalit included three stages, described in the following sections.

Programme Development

A national interdisciplinary team was established; its members were professionals from the fields of health promotion, family medicine, diabetology, nursing, nutrition, and service marketing. The team assessed and defined needs and developed the strategy for the intervention programme.

Focus groups with community members supported the efforts for needs assessment and planning. Additionally, the team developed culturally appropriate health promotion tools on the topics of eating habits, physical activity, smoking cessation, self-monitoring, and self-care.

Programme Implementation

The initial programme was conducted during the period 2001–2003; it focused on healthy lifestyles for the entire family and was open to the entire local community living in Israeli Arab towns and villages, not only diabetics. Lectures and group discussions were conducted with community health professionals, and individual lifestyle consultations were conducted on relevant topics. All health information and instruction in the community events included Arabic written material and pictograms that were distributed to participants. Over 6,000 residents from over 20 communities participated in the programme.

Evaluation Results and Conclusions

The programme's impact and outcome evaluation was conducted by telephone interviews among a representative sample of the participants; it examined the following indicators: change in health behaviour, attitudes toward diabetes, satisfaction with the programme, and change in hemoglobin A1C (HbA1C). The evaluation showed that the event significantly contributed to reported behaviour change among the participants. Diabetes control measured by HbA1C levels among programme participants showed a significant increase in the percentage of participants whose measures improved. Similar improvements were not observed in the comparison population.

The recommendations derived from the findings from the initiative were:

1) A need for in-depth community programmes, above and beyond community events.
2) Expressed interest in ongoing health promotion lifestyle and chronic disease prevention interventions.
3) The primary care clinic was noted as an appropriate setting for health promotion events, particularly regarding chronic disease prevention.

4)   Individual lifestyle counselling was recommended as part of the community initiative as well as in-depth behaviour change workshops.

All of the above-mentioned recommendations were henceforth applied in Clalit's national diabetes programme strategy, emphasizing health literacy, self-management, and maintenance.

CONCLUSION

The health literacy of communities has gained more international and local attention by public health and primary care health services, particularly with regard to needs based on culture and ethnicity. Such communities and especially cultures in transition, from traditional to western, are demonstrating poorer health indicators. Confronted with unfamiliar environmental, social, economic, and physical resources for maintaining and improving health, traditional communities are at significantly higher risk for chronic disease; at the same time, local health and social services are often unprepared for meeting these challenges in a culturally appropriate way.

This chapter has reviewed some examples of research and practice that are contributing to the body of knowledge regarding what is needed, what succeeds, and what does not. The examples above, whilst illustrating different approaches, show that community-based approaches using advocacy and the mediation of health care systems are more likely to be effective than those that neglect to involve the community in planning and implementation. Health should be addressed not only *in* or *with* communities but in complete partnership with communities, adopting models such as the Community Participatory Action for Health model for involving communities (Masude, Creighton, Nixon, and Frankish, 2011). These examples of best practice display the value of lasting partnerships not only for sustainable practice in health literacy and promotion but also for using participative methods in data gathering on a more equitable and culturally appropriate basis for working to improve health in the community.

Questions for Reflection

1)   How can community empowerment promote functional, critical, and interactive literacy?

2) How are health literacy and cultural competence related in the community context?
3) What is the role of the members of the community in understanding health needs and promoting health literacy?
4) To what extent is functional literacy necessary for communities to participate in the promotion of health?

REFERENCES

American Medical Association Ad Hoc Committee on Health Literacy. (1999). Health literacy: Report of the Council of Scientific Affairs, American Medical Association. *Journal of the American Medical Association, 281*(6), 552-557.

Baker, D. W., Wolf, M. S., Feinglass, J., Thompson, J. A., Gazmararian, J. A., and Huang, J. (2007). Health literacy and mortality among elderly persons. *Archives of Internal Medicine, 167*(14), 1503-1509. doi:<p>10.1001/archinte.167.14.1503</p>.

Barrera-Anderson, T., Olives, T., Larsen, K., and Pereira, A. (2007). Health literacy in native Spanish-speaking immigrants in Minneapolis. *Travel Medicine and Infectious Disease, 5*(6), 410.

Begoray, D. L., Wharf-Higgins, J., and MacDonald, M. (2009). High school health curriculum and health literacy: Canadian student voices. *Global Health Promotion, 16*(4), 35-42.

Betancourt, J. R., Green, A. R., and Carrillo, J. E. (2002). *Cultural competence in health care: Emerging frameworks and practical approaches.* New York, NY: The Commonwealth Fund.

Cabinet Office. (2010, May). *Building the Big Society* (briefing note). Retrieved from http://www.cabinetoffice.gov.uk/news/building-big-society.

Cameron, D. (2011). *Radicalisation and Islamic extremism.* Retrieved from http://www.number10.gov.uk/news/pms-speech-at-munich-security-conference/.

Canadian Public Health Association. (2006). *Health literacy interventions.* Ottawa, Canada: Author. Retrieved from http://www.cpha.ca/uploads/portals/h-l/interventions_e.pdf.

Cemlyn, S., Greenfields, M., Burnett, S., Matthews, Z., and Whitwell, C. (2009). *Inequalities experienced by Gypsy and Traveller communities: A review.* Manchester, England: Equality and Human Rights Commission.

Chinn, D. (2011). Critical health literacy: A review and critical analysis. *Social Science and Medicine, 73*, 60-67.

Epstein, L. (2006). *Reducing health inequality and health inequity in Israel: Towards a national policy and action programme – summary report.* Jerusalem, Israel: Smokler Center for Policy Research, Myers–JDC–Brookdale Institute.

Eysenbach, G., Powell, J., Englesakis, M., Rizo, C., and Stern, A. (2004). Health related virtual communities and electronic support groups: Systematic review of the effects of online peer to peer interactions. *British Medical Journal, 328,* 1166-1172.

Foster, G. (1978). *Medical anthropology.* New York, NY: John Wiley.

Fox, S. (2011). *The social life of health information, 2011.* Washington, DC: Pew Research Center's Internet and American Life Project. Retrieved from http://pewinternet.org/~/media//Files/Reports/2011/PIP_Social_Life_of_Health_Info.pdf.

Freedman, D. A., Bess, K. D., Tucker, H. A., Boyd, D. L., Tuchman, A. M., and Wallston, K. A. (2009). Public health literacy defined. *American Journal of Preventive Medicine, 36*(5), 446-451.

Freire, P. (1970). *Pedagogy of the oppressed.* New York, NY: Seabury.

Gazmararian, J. A., Williams, M. V., Peel, J., and Baker, D. W. (2003). Health literacy and knowledge of chronic disease. *Patient Education and Counseling, 51*(3), 267–275.

Goldracht, M., Levin, D., Peled, O., Poraz, I., Stern, E., Brami, J. L., ... Dreiner, J. (2011). Twelve-year follow-up of a population-based primary care diabetes program in Israel. *International Journal for Quality in Health Care.* Advance online publication. doi:10.1093/intqhc/mzr051.

Hoebel, E. A., and Frost, E. L. (1976). *Cultural and social anthropology.* New York, NY: McGraw-Hill.

Hossain, P., Kawar, B., and El Nahas, M. (2007). Obesity and diabetes in the developing world — A growing challenge. *New England Journal of Medicine, 356*(3), 213-215.

Jahan, R. A. (2000). Promoting health literacy: A case study in the prevention of diarroheal disease from Bangladesh. *Health Promotion International, 15*(4), 285-291.

Kagawa-Singer, M. (2011). Impact of culture on health outcomes. *Journal of Pediatric Hematologic Oncology, 33*, S90–S95.

Kickbusch, I. S. (2001). Health literacy: Addressing the health and education divide. *Health Promotion International, 16*(3), 289-297.

King, J. (2007). *Environmental scan of interventions to improve health literacy: Final report.* Antigonish, Canada: National Collaborating Centre for Determinants of Health. Retrieved from http://www.nccdh.ca/ supportfiles/NCCDH_EnvScanLiteracy_Sep909.pdf.

Kintsch, W. (1998). *Comprehension: A paradigm for cognition.* Cambridge, MA: Cambridge University Press.

Kreps, G. L., and Sparks, L. (2008). Meeting the health literacy needs of immigrant populations. *Patient Education and Counseling, 71*(3), 328-332.

Kutner, M., Greenberg, E., Jin, Y., and Paulsen, C. (2006). *The health literacy of America's adults: Results from the 2003 National Assessment of Adult Literacy.* Washington, DC: National Center for Education Statistics. Available fromhttp://nces.ed.gov/pubsearch/pubsinfo.asp?pubid=2006483.

Lalonde, M. (1974). *A new perspective on the health of Canadians.* Ottawa, Canada: Ministry of National Health and Welfare.

Levin, D. (1980). *Western and traditional medical systems: Paradigms, interaction and change.* Unpublished manuscript. Tufts University, Medford, MA.

Levin-Zamir, D., Keret, S., Yaakovson, O., Lev, B., Kay, C., and Verber, G. (2011). Refuah Shlema: A cross-cultural programme for promoting communication and health among Ethiopian immigrants in the primary health care setting in Israel. *Global Health Promotion, 18*(1), 51-54.

Levin-Zamir, D., Lemish, D., and Gofin, R. (2011). Media health literacy (MHL): Development and measurement of the concept among adolescents. *Health Education Research, 26*(2), 323-335.

Levin-Zamir, D., Lipsky, D., Goldberg, E., and Melamud, T. (1993). Health education for Ethiopian immigrants in Israel, 1991–1992. *Israel Journal of Medical Sciences, 29*, 422-428.

Masude, J. R., Creighton, M. A., Nixon, S., and Frankish, F. (2011). Building capacity for community-based participatory research for health disparities in Canada: The case of "Partnerships in Community Health Research." *Health Promotion Practice, 12*(2), 280-292.

National Institute for Health and Clinical Excellence. (2008). *Community engagement to improve health.* London, England: Author.

National Primary Care Research and Development Centre. (2006). *The national evaluation of the pilot phase of the Expert Patient Programme: Final report.* Manchester, England: Author.

Naidoo, J., and Wills, J. (2010). *Developing practice for public health and health promotion.* London, England: Balliere Tindall.

Nielsen-Bohlman, L., Panzer, A. M., and Kindig, D. A. (Eds.). (2004). *Health literacy: A prescription to end confusion.* Washington, DC: Institute of Medicine of the National Academies and The National Academies Press.

Nirel, N., Rosen, B., and Ismail, S. (2000). *'Refuah Shlema': An intervention programme for Ethiopian immigrants in primary care clinics: Results of an evaluation study.* Jerusalem, Israel: Smokler Center for Policy Research and Myers–JDC–Brookdale Institute.

Nova Scotia Department of Health. (2010). *Messages for all voices: Integrating cultural competence and health literacy in health materials, forms, and signage.* Halifax, Canada: Province of Nova Scotia. Available from http://www.gov.ns.ca/health/primaryhealthcare/documents/messages %20for%20all%20voices-%20full%20length%20tool.pdf.

Nutbeam, D. (2000). Health literacy as a public health goal: A challenge for contemporary health education and communication strategies into the 21st century. *Health Promotion International, 15*(3), 259-267.

Nutbeam, D. (2008). The evolving concept of health literacy. *Social Science and Medicine, 67*(12), 2072-2078.

Papen, U. (2009). Literacy, learning and health: A social practices view of health literacy. *Literacy and Numeracy Studies, 16*(2), 19-35.

Parikh, N. S., Parker, R. M., Nurss, J. R., Baker, D. W, and Williams, M. V. (1996). Shame and health literacy: The unspoken connection. *Patient Education and Counselling, 27*(1), 33 39.

Parry, G., Van Cleemput, P., Peters, J., Walters, S., Thomas, K., and Cooper, C. (2004). Health status of Gypsies and Travellers in England. *Journal of Epidemiology and Community Health, 61*, 198-204.

Pleasant, A., and Kuruvilla, S. (2008). A tale of two health literacies: Public health and clinical approaches to health literacy. *Health Promotion International, 23*(2), 152-159. doi:10.1093/heapro/dan001.

Porr, C., Drummond, J., and Richter, S. (2006). Health literacy as an empowerment tool for low-income mothers. *Family and Community Health, 29*(4), 328-335.

Poureslami, I. M., Rootman, I., Balka, E., Devarakonda, R., Hatch, J., and Fitzgerald, J. M. (2007). A systematic review of asthma and health literacy: A cultural-ethnic perspective in Canada. *Medscape General Medicine, 9*(3), 40.

Simich, L. (2009). *Health literacy and immigrant populations* (Policy brief to Public Health Agency of Canada and Metropolis Canada). Toronto, Canada: Author. Available from http://canada.metropolis.net/pdfs/health_ literacy_policy_brief_jun15_e.pdf.

Smart, H., Titterton, M., and Clark, C. (2003). A literature review of the health of Gypsy/Traveller families in Scotland: The challenges for health promotion. *Health Education, 103*(3), 156-165.

Sudore, R. L., Yaffe, K., Satterfield, S., Harris, T. B., Mehta, K. M., Simonsick, E. M., ... Schillinger, D. (2006). Limited literacy and mortality in the elderly: The health, aging, and body composition study. *Journal of General Internal Medicine, 21*(8), 806-812. doi:10.1111/j.1525-1497.2006.00539.x.

Sussex Traveller Women's Health Project. (n.d.). *Friends, families and travellers: Final project report 2003-2006.* East Sussex, England: Author. Available from http://www.gypsy-traveller.org/pdfs/health_annual_report_05.pdf.

Thomson, M. D., and Hoffman-Goetz, L. (2011). Application of the health literacy framework to diet-related cancer prevention conversations of older immigrant women to Canada. *Health Promotion International.* Advance online publication. doi:10.1093/heapro/dar019.

United States Department of Health and Human Services. (2000a). *Healthy people 2010: Understanding and improving health.* Washington, DC: Author.

United States Department of Health and Human Services, Office of Minority Health. (2000b). *Assuring cultural competence in health care: Recommendations for national standards and outcomes-focused research agenda.* Washington, DC: US Government Printing Office.

United States Institute of Medicine. (2002). *Speaking of health.* Washington, DC: The National Academies Press.

Useem, J., Useem, R., and Donoghue, J. (1963). Men in the middle of the third culture: The roles of American and non-Western people in cross-cultural administration. *Human Organization, 22*(3), 169-179.

Van Cleemput, P. (2008). *Gypsies and Travellers accessing primary health care: Interactions with health staff and requirements for 'culturally safe' services* (Unpublished doctoral dissertation). University of Sheffield, Sheffield, England.

Van Cleemput, P., Thomas, K., Parry, G., Peters, J., and Cooper, C. (2007). The health-related beliefs and experience of Gypsies and Travellers: A qualitative study. *Journal of Epidemiology and Community Health, 61*, 205-210.

Wang, R. (2000). Critical health literacy: A case study from China in schistosomiasis control. *Health Promotion International, 15*(3), 269-274.

World Health Organization. (1986). *Ottawa charter for health promotion.* Geneva, Switzerland.

World Health Organization. (1998). *Health promotion glossary.* Geneva, Switzerland.

Zamora, H., and Clingerman, E. M. (2011). Health literacy among older adults: A systematic literature review. *Journal of Gerontological Nursing, 37*(10), 32-40. doi:10.3928/00989134-20110503-02.

Zanchetta, M. S., and Poureslami, I. M. (2006). Health literacy within the reality of immigrants' culture and language. *Canadian Journal of Public Health, 97*(S2), S26-30. Available from http://journal.cpha.ca/index.php/cjph/articlc/view/1523/1712.

In: Health Literacy in Context   ISBN: 978-1-61942-921-5
Eds.: D.Begoray, D.Gillis, G.Rowlands © 2012 Nova Science Publishers, Inc.

Chapter 7

HEALTH LITERACY: AN ECONOMIC PERSPECTIVE

Diarmuid Coughlan *

ABSTRACT

A presentation at a 2009 Institute of Medicine health literacy workshop provides a conceptual framework to discuss the various economic angles of health literacy. To date, much of the research has focused on the skills and abilities of individuals with little attention paid to the other side of the *health literacy coin*—the demands/complexities of the health care system. This chapter examines both sides of the coin and uses the English health care system as a case study to illustrate an economic perspective of health literacy. The following questions are considered: Are health-literate individuals more efficient users of health care resources? Can we produce better health through investing in health literacy? Do health literacy interventions improve one's health outcomes? How does a third-party payer view health literacy? What incentive is there for a provider to advocate health literacy principles? How should a policy maker approach health literacy? The author concludes that it is imperative that the economic data requirements for decision making are understood and embraced by health literacy advocates.

* E-mail: dcoughla@jhsph.edu or diarmuidcoughlan@hotmail.com.

INTRODUCTION

The aim of this chapter is to give readers a primer on how the economic perspective may influence the health care decision-making process. In turn, the hope is to strengthen the advocacy argument in lobbying decision makers to support evidence-based health literacy initiatives. Reference to the advocacy community in this chapter encompasses a wide range of people from academic researchers to practitioners (e.g., adult educators, health professionals) and lay caregivers; the common link is that, as advocates, they all seek resources and implementation of their health literacy-themed research, interventions, and applications.

Economics is the study of choice when resources (e.g., skilled labour, hospital beds, money, time) are scarce. When operating under budget constraints and/or health targets, multiple decisions have to be made about how to use these resources in expectation of deriving the greatest net benefit (Stinnett and Mullahy, 1998). The true economic cost of delivering health care is known as the *opportunity cost*; alternatively, it can be viewed as *health benefits forgone*. To help quantify choices faced by decision makers, the economic cost of forgone health benefits is most often represented in monetary terms.

The use of economic evaluation principles as a decision-making tool is seen as an explicit, transparent mechanism in many jurisdictions. Numerous governments (e.g., Australia, Canada, the United Kingdom [UK]) have devolved responsibility to expert-led agencies, often called health technology assessment (HTA) agencies, to conduct economic evaluations of health care interventions and to make coverage and reimbursement decisions (Hutton et al., 2006). Health literacy advocates need to be cognizant of these organisations, especially their evidence criteria and decision rules. In times of austerity, it is imperative that health literacy initiatives show their value explicitly.

The term *health literacy* has come to mean different things to various audiences and is a source of considerable confusion and debate (Baker, 2006). From an economic analyst's perspective, it makes the job of evaluating health literacy initiatives even more daunting. Parker (2009) provided a useful conceptual framework (Figure 1) to discuss the various economic angles of health literacy: "One must align skills and abilities [of individuals] with the demands and complexity of the system. When that is accomplished, one has health literacy." (p. 92).

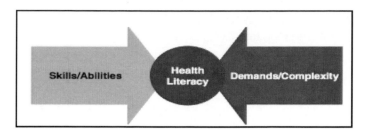

Figure 1. Health literacy framework (Parker, 2009. Reprinted with permission).

This framework allows the economic considerations of health literacy to be divided in terms of the individual and the health care system. Although the majority of research on health literacy has been aimed at improving the skills or abilities of individuals, influencing decision makers to lessen the demands on individuals may prove to be a more effective strategy. Realizing efficiency gains is the aspiration for many decision makers on the other side of the *health literacy coin* (Kirsch, Roter, Pisano, and King, 2010). Incorporating an economic argument is one tool that can help decision makers accomplish this goal.

This chapter is divided into three parts. The first part discusses the health literacy skills and abilities of the individual by outlining the estimated costs of low health literacy, highlighting pertinent theory, and commenting upon interventions aimed at improving the skills of certain population groups. The second part examines the demands and complexities of the health literacy framework by outlining the overall costs of low health literacy to the health care system. Interwovenly, the perspectives of payers, providers, and policy makers are considered. The third part provides an economic perspective on health literacy in England as an example of a jurisdiction with a HTA agency, the National Institute of Health and Clinical Excellence (NICE).

SKILLS AND ABILITIES OF THE INDIVIDUAL

Fuchs (1974/1998) stated that, "The greatest potential for improving health lies in what we do and don't do for ourselves. The choice is ours." (p. 55). The often-cited definition of health literacy—"the degree to which individuals have the capacity to obtain, process, and understand basic health information and services needed to make appropriate health decisions" (Ratzan and Parker, 2000, p. 3)—galvanizes the assertion that an individual's

health literacy skills are part of the building blocks in achieving Fuchs'
philosophical position on improving health.

Given full information and opportunity, one would assume that
individuals act rationally and adopt healthy behaviours. Unfortunately, this is
not always the case. The key issue should be whether an individual is fully
informed on the choices to be made; if so, then truly the choice is their own.
Economists refer to the information asymmetry that exists between the
informed principal (i.e., doctor) and the agent (i.e., patient). From this
perspective, health literacy is essentially about closing the gap between the
principal and the agent. Economists are preoccupied with choice; they instruct
policy makers to *nudge* individuals to make healthier choices. All in all, this
approach is intended to avoid the consequences of poor choices that result in
greater health costs and negative externalities upon the wider society.
Economists refer to an externality or transaction spillover as a cost or benefit,
not transmitted through prices, incurred by a party who did not agree to the
action causing the cost or benefit. An example of a negative externality is
passive smoke.

Pleasant and Kuruvilla (2008) posited that the conceptualisation of health
literacy has evolved into two main approaches: public health and clinical. This
division suggests that the general public can be thought of in two distinct ways
reflective of their health literacy roles: as individuals (members of the public)
or as patients (users of health services). A key goal in public health policy is to
enable individuals to make informed decisions about adopting healthy
behaviours to live better quality lives, preventing unhealthy and self-inflicted
conditions such as obesity and related conditions (e.g., Type 2 diabetes
mellitus and coronary heart disease). From a clinical perspective, the goal of
health literacy would be to help patients requiring health services to become
more efficient users of the health care system.

Individuals are described in the literature as having low, below basic,
inadequate, basic, functional, intermediate, adequate, or proficient health
literacy. These terms are specific to the context and to the measurement tool
used. Such terms underline the lack of standardisation in the field, thus making
comparison of the burden of low health literacy across populations difficult.
Pleasant (2009) noted that screening and measuring are two distinct activities.
Screening tools (e.g., Rapid Estimate in Adult Literacy in Medicine
[REALM]) are often used as proxy measurement tools; as such, this is the rate-
limiting step in facilitating economic analyses of the impact of low health
literacy. Individual health literacy is a matter of applying skills and abilities to
meet demands imposed by situations that are evolving along the lifecycle.

Viewed in this way, health literacy is rendered a measureless concept; thus, its economic impact is impossible to quantify.

The Challenge in Measuring Individual Cost/Resource Utilisation in Health Literacy Studies

Only a few studies, all from the United States, have looked at the cost/resource utilisation of those deemed to have limited health literacy compared to those with adequate health literacy (Table 1). It should be noted that the sample population and the outcome measures reported are quite diverse in these studies. Moreover, as Eichler, Wieser, and Brügger (2009) noted in their systematic review, the cost studies varied widely in methodological quality and none of the studies considered indirect costs (e.g., mortality costs, time lost from work, decreased productivity from/at work).

Table 1. Studies Reporting Cost/resource Utilisation by Health Literacy Level

Author(s); Year; Country	Sample population	Outcome measure	Main results
Sanders, Thompson, and Wilkinson; 2007; USA	Caregivers of children	Use of child health services	Adequate HL vs. low HL $1514.74 vs. 1657.90 Not a SS diference based on HL
Howard, Gazmararian, and Parker; 2005; USA	Medicare managed care enrollees	Medical costs	ER: Δ$108 (SS) I/P: Δ$1543 (MSS) TC: Δ$596 (Not SS) Inefficient mix of HC services consumed by enrollees with low HL
Weiss and Palmer; 2004; USA	Medically needy and indigent Medicaid	Health care costs	Adequate HL vs. low HL $2,891/year vs. $10,688/year Very small study ($n = 74$). Limited reading skills associated with greater HC charges.

Note. ER = emergency room; HC = health care; HL = health literacy; I/P = inpatient; MSS = marginally statistically significant; SS = statistically significant; TC = total cost; Δ = incremental difference between adequate and low HL individuals.

Technical methodological (econometric) issues persist in the analysis of costing data. For example, medical spending data are often highly skewed, implying that the variance is large relative to the mean. So, results using mean costs may not give a complete picture. Additionally, in order to make robust estimates of costs attributable to one's health literacy level, the issue of confounding must be considered. Cho, Lee, Arozullah, and Crittenden (2008) conducted path analyses, which focuses on examining the web of relationships among measured variables, to examine the effects of health literacy on health status and health care utilisation while controlling for obvious confounders (i.e., gender, race, education attainment); whereas Bennett, Chen, Soroui, and White (2009) discussed confounding and mediating effects associated with the health literacy variable and preventive health behaviours. Therefore, accounting for the channels through which health literacy affects health care utilisation is important to any economic analysis. Several conceptual models exist that link health literacy to health outcomes (Baker, 2006; McCormack, 2009), health status (Osborn, Paasche-Orlow, Bailey, and Wolf, 2011), and health care resource utilisation (Paasche-Orlow and Wolf, 2007). Methodological issues aside, recent research has shed some light on key questions pertaining to the economics of individual health literacy.

Are Health-Literate People More Efficient Users of Health Care Resources?

The hypothesis that an individual with an adequate health literacy level would be a more efficient user of health care resources is essentially an empirical question. In monetary terms, three US studies (Table 1) reported that patients with limited health literacy incurred additional health care expenditures in the range of $143–7,798 per person per year than people with adequate health literacy level. This is a wide range explained by the sample population, the length of follow-up, and the context of how the costing data were collected. Howard, Gazmararian, and Parker (2005) suggested how estimates could be improved:

> Very large sample sizes are needed to precisely identify differences in spending between health literacy groups … inclusion of health literacy measures in large population surveys such as the National Health Interview Survey or the Medicare Current Beneficiary Survey, would allow researchers to estimate attributable costs more precisely in the future. (p. 376)

Longitudinal studies could provide a wonderful opportunity to look at resource use based on an individual's health literacy ability (caveat: a standardized measure of one's health literacy ability be used in the surveys). It would allow an individual's health literacy ability to be considered as a separate variable to education attainment. Baker et al. (2007) used reading fluency as a proxy for health literacy and determined it to be a more powerful variable than education for examining the association between socioeconomic status and health. The US evidence does suggest that more health-literate individuals are more efficient users of health care resources than those with limited health literacy (Berkman et al. 2011).

Can We Produce Good Health through Better Health Literacy?

One of the most influential theoretical models in health economics is the Grossman (1972) demand for health model, which predicts that individuals with more education and health knowledge unambiguously demand more health. However, the model is ambiguous in predicting a more educated person's derived demand for preventative health care. Educated individuals either demand and utilize more preventative health care because they are investing in their health stock or demand and utilize less preventative health care because they are more efficient users of the preventative health care already received. This concept of producing good health by investing in one's self is termed *health capital production* and was introduced by Grossman through his seminal research designed to show how individuals make decisions about their health. This conceptual model assumes that health literacy in combination with other factors (e.g., education, income, gender) affects an individual's ability to essentially produce health, that is, to stay healthy. The model also assumes that the demand for medical care is one ingredient that produces health and, thus, depends on health literacy (Vernon, Trujillo, Rosenbaum, and DeBuono, 2007).

Grossman (1972) also introduced the idea of health as an investment in human capital. From an economic rationale, individuals are able to increase their human capital in later years by investing presently in health. An individual can view being health literate as an investment that will bring about a better quality of life in the future. However, empirical research has found that individuals rationally reduce their use of preventive care as their period of payoffs to the original investment in care shortens over their lifecycle (Kenkel, 1994). As such, one is less likely to invest or consume preventative health care as one ages; for example, the value of a mammogram is considerably less to an 85-year-old woman than to a 55-year-old woman. In addition, Kenkel (1994) found that schooling is an important determinant of demand, with more educated people much more likely to use preventive services.

In their study of preventive health care use among US Medicare enrolees in a managed care organisation, Scott, Gazmararian, Williams, and Baker (2002) found that inadequate health literacy is independently associated with lower use of preventive health services (e.g., having an influenza or pneumococcal vaccination or a Papanicolaou smear cervical cancer screening test). Also, these female patients were less likely in the previous two years to have had a mammogram when compared to patients with adequate health literacy. Interestingly however, Smith et al. (2010) found in a randomized control trial in Australia that decision support aids resulted in more informed treatment group but had a lower uptake of bowel cancer screening.

Wolf, Gazmararian, and Baker (2007) found that limited health literacy was not significantly associated with health-risk behaviours (e.g., self-reported cigarette smoking, alcohol consumption, physical activity, body mass index, and seat belt use). The older age profile (65+ years) of the patients in these studies limits the generalisability of these results but is consistent with Kenkel's (1994) empirical work. Note that in the US health care setting, confounding factors such as health insurance status and an individual's ability to pay can greatly affect an individual's use of preventive health care services. The new US health care reform law (Patient Protection and Affordable Care Act of 2010) seeks to improve coverage of prevention benefits. Medicare will cover a free, annual, comprehensive wellness visit and personalized prevention plan (see http://www.kff.org/healthreform/7948.cfm for a summary of key changes to Medicare).

Where access to health services is available to all, an individual's health literacy status is a likely indicator of whether an individual actually chooses to use such preventive health care services. Individuals have the potential to achieve or maintain good health though better health literacy. The onus is on the advocacy community to design interventions that demonstrate empirically to policy makers the channels through which health literacy produces better health; hopefully, such interventions will be cost-saving.

Do Health Literacy Interventions Improve Health Outcomes?

Clement, Ibrahim, Crichton, Wolf, and Rowlands (2009) conducted a systematic review of complex interventions aimed at improving the health of people with limited literacy; the interventions included nutrition action plans (Howard-Pitney, Winkleby, Albright, Bruce, and Fortmann, 1997), a medication adherence program (van Servellen et al., 2005), and a health failure self-management program (DeWalt et al., 2006). The review authors stated that, "Methodological short-comings and the mixed nature of some of the findings indicate that interventions would most appropriately be introduced in an evaluative or research context" (p. 350). The updated systematic review of low health literacy and health outcomes prepared for the US Agency for Healthcare Research and Quality noted that among intervention studies (27 randomized controlled trials [RCTs], 2 cluster RCTs, and 13 quasi-experimental designs) the strength of evidence for specific design features was low or insufficient (Berkman et al., 2011).

Interventions aimed at individuals are educational and managerial in nature; hence, the two classes of outcome most likely to improve were individuals' health knowledge and self-efficacy. However, decision makers often need to consider the size of clinical changes because some interventions are highly resource-intensive. Though an intervention may be efficacious in a clinical trial setting, will it be effective in a real world setting? And, subsequently, will it represent value-for-money? It would be informative to decision makers to incorporate an economic evaluation to future health literacy intervention studies.

Further economic perspective research could study the importance of skills training to an individual by using a willingness-to-pay approach. As people from lower socioeconomic status are disproportionately affected by low health literacy, what incentives can a clinician, insurance company, or government make to entice an individual to partake in a proven health literacy intervention?

DEMANDS AND COMPLEXITIES OF THE HEALTH CARE SYSTEM

The other side of the health literacy framework coin is the health care system. This side can be considered to be composed of three distinct groups:

payers, providers, and policy makers. All three groups are faced with the similar dilemma of obtaining value for the money for which they are responsible for. Establishing the nature and burden of low health literacy is often required before addressing it.

Eichler et al. (2009) reported that (a) the prevalence of limited health literacy is considerable (range 34–59%) and (b) on the health system level the additional cost of limited health literacy ranges from 3 to 5% of the total health care cost per year. A summary of the literature that has estimated the cost of low health literacy per year and the estimated percentage of health care costs attributed to low health literacy in various jurisdictions is presented in Table 2. Essentially, two slightly differing calculating methods have been used to make estimates concerning the cost of low health literacy on the health care system (Vernon, Trujillo, Rosenbaum et al., 2007; Wieser, Moschetti, Eichler, Holly, and Brügger, 2008).

Table 2. System-level Costs of Low Health Literacy

Country; State	Year	Estimated cost of low HL (per year)	Estimated % of HC expenditure due to low HL	Author(s) (year); Funding source
USA	1998	$30–73bn	3.2–7.6%	Friedland (1998)
	2002	$32–58bn		NAAS—U.S. Congress
USA	2007	$106–238bn	7–17%	Vernon, Trujillo, Rosenbaum, and DeBuono (2007) NBER
USA; Missouri	2007	$3.3–7.5bn	n/r	Vernon, Trujilo, and Keener Hughen (2007) MFH—HLM
USA; Wisconsin	2009	$3.4–7.6bn	n/r	Vernon (2009) Wisconsin Literacy Inc.
USA; Iowa	2011	$1.9–4.2bn	n/r	Health Literacy Iowa (n.d.) Iowa Health System
Switzerland	2006	CHF 1.5bn ($1.4bn)	3%	Spycher (2006) BASS
Switzerland	2008	CHF 2.279bn ($2.1bn)	4.3%	Wieser, Moschetti, Eichler, Holly, and Brügger (2008)
		CHF 4.772bn ($4.4bn)	9.1%	IEMS—HPS

Note. NAAS = National Academy on an Aging Society; NBER = National Bureau of Economic Research; MFH = Missouri Foundation for Health; HLM = Health Literacy Missouri; BASS = Buro fur Arbeits und Sozialpolitische Studien; IEMS = Institute of Health Economics and Management (University of Lausanne and Zurich); HPS = Health Promotion Switzerland; n/r = not reported.

Typically in health care, close coordination over time and within care episodes improves both health outcomes and efficiency. Close coordination is problematic in the highly fragmented US health care system because the financing and delivery of care is distributed across a variety of distinct and often competing entities—each with its own objectives, obligations, and capabilities (Cebul, Rebitzer, Taylor, and Votruba, 2008). This is in turn problematic to making inferences about the true cost of low health literacy in the US. Vernon, Trujillo, Rosenbaum et al. (2007) stated:

> Our intent is to approximate only the order of magnitude of the economic costs of low health literacy in the U.S. The value of such approximations is for just this purpose: to raise awareness of the relative size and magnitude of the economic costs involved. It is from this perspective and within this context only, that our estimates might be considered. (p. 6)

They cited the need for individual-level data in order to make more robust estimates of the costs and especially to estimate the proportion of health care expenditures attributable to low functional literacy and the proportion attributable to other factors (covariates).

In Switzerland, health insurance is universal and compulsory for all residents; it can be supplemented by private, complementary insurance policies that cover some treatment categories not included in the basic insurance. Wieser et al. (2008) stated:

> The most important limitation of our exercise is the lack of information on the relationship between limited health literacy and healthcare costs in Switzerland.... Ideally this analysis would be based on a representative sample of the population including micro (=patient level) data on healthcare costs, health literacy and health conditions. (p. 28)

The Swiss economic model uses input variables extrapolated from US data (Howard et al., 2005) and is an extension of the cost model proposed by the US researchers. The bottom line is that both groups of researchers use the best available population data to make estimates of the cost of low health literacy to their health care system.

Perhaps what is inhibiting estimating the cost of low health literacy the most remains that an acceptable measurement tool of health literacy does not exist. Therefore, what is needed is a tool that can link an individual's health literacy status with their health conditions and, subsequently, their health care costs. Establishing accurately the financial burden of low health literacy is useful information for payers asked to reimburse health literacy-themed interventions.

How Does a Third-Party Payer View Health Literacy?

The limited evidence suggests that the central issue for third-party payers (e.g., health insurers and publicly funded health care systems) is that individuals who do not understand and cannot act on the medical information and instructions are likely to be more costly. Fundamentally, the principle of health insurance is essentially a form of risk management against incurring medical expenses. Therefore, it makes economic sense that individuals be *nudged* by third-party payers into proactively making healthy lifestyle decisions in a bid to avoid reactive medical care procedures and charges.

For the private health insurers, efficiency gains, cost containment, and profit are the paramount attributes to making decisions about how to package a health insurance plan. However, under health care reform, US insurers will be required to produce *coverage fact labels*. The law directed the National Association of Insurance Commissioners to draft these labels. Consumers shopping for a health care policy can compare the costs and coverage of different plans and make the appropriate choices. Examples for three medical conditions (i.e., maternity care, diabetes, and breast cancer) are available (see http://www.kaiserhealthnews.   org/stories/2011/may/05/documents-health-insurance-coverage-labels.aspx).

The July 2011 IOM workshop entitled *Facilitating State Health Exchange Communication through the Use of Health Literate Practices* highlighted the problems individuals have understanding insurance jargon and the public's knowledge about supplemental out-of-pocket costs, benefits coverage, and entitlements. It should be noted that America's Health Insurance Plans have created a task force on health literacy. An example of their commitment to the easing of the demands placed upon individuals is a checklist of reader- and user-friendly web design for health plans. These are encouraging signs in helping consumers navigate the health care system; insurers may see a reduction in unnecessary costs.

In a public health care setting, similar economic aspirations exist with the added dimension of equity. Hasnain-Wynia and Wolf (2010) considered the case of health literacy as the missing link in the efforts to redress inequities in health care. Moreover, in jurisdictions that use HTA agencies for health care resource allocation of public funds, equity is an important consideration in decision making, hence the use of economic evaluations. The health literacy research community needs to be cognizant of HTA agency requirements regarding the acceptable methodology of economic evaluations and how that agency deems an intervention to be cost-effective. To date, there are no reported cost-effectiveness studies on any health literacy-themed interventions (Eichler et al., 2009).

Be they public or private, third-party payers are likely to view health literacy as a remedy to unnecessary costs among individuals. Payers must also entice providers into advocating health literacy principles to deliver value-driven health care.

What Incentive Is There for Providers to Advocate Health Literacy Principles?

Aligning the incentive structure such that providers interact with patients in a health literacy manner would be an interesting proposal. An example of an incentive mechanism is the physician pay-for-performance scheme operational in the UK and the US. In the US setting, patient education is not part of the remuneration scheme and, as such, is not promoted by current pay-for-performance programs. Volandes and Paasche-Orlow (2007), well-known health literacy advocates, proposed a shift of quality measures away from items such as laboratory tests toward patient education. Developing clear communication strategies may indeed improve patients' health outcomes, but would a policy that involves remuneration based on improving patient education be good use of a policy makers' limited budget?

Another quality indicator aimed at US health care organisations may arise from the Consumer Assessment of Healthcare Providers and Systems (CAHPS) surveys that measure system demands and complexity. CAHPS is a set of standardised, evidence-based surveys for assessing patients' experiences with their health care encounters. The project has started to develop reports that can be used by providers (e.g., hospitals, primary care clinics) to identify areas for quality improvement (Weider Ocampo, 2009). If providers receive funding based on their quality performance, surveys such as CAHPS will have great importance to health care managers due to their financial links.

From an economic perspective, will the payers of these schemes/policies get the anticipated *bang for their buck*? Or will it be a costly, incentive-based strategy that providers can *game* with negative, unintended consequences? The devil is in the details of such schemes and policies.

How Should a Policy Maker Approach Health Literacy?

The audience for many advocates is an appropriate policy maker—be they at the local, regional, or national level. One of the most fundamental questions regarding health literacy is: How the term should be framed?- Should it be viewed as a health inequality, social disparity, or a public health issue? These approaches motivate the topic differently and impact upon the economic perspective.

In the White Paper *Together for Health: A Strategic Approach for the EU 2008-2013*, the European Commission (2007) refers to the promotion of health literacy as one of the key actions to reduce health inequalities within the EU. In England, under the Labour government (1997–2010), the Department of Health considered health literacy as part of its health inequalities strategy (Department of Health, England [DHE], 2008).

By promoting a shared health literacy and health disparities (inequalities) research agenda, Paasche-Orlow and Wolf (2010) noted that in a number of US studies (Osborn et al., 2011; Osborn, Paasche-Orlow, Davis, and Wolf, 2007; Volandes and Paasche-Orlow, 2007) completely different conclusions would have been made without concurrent evaluation of race and health literacy.

Fundamentally, on what basis can health literacy be considered a health inequality? Taking a social justice perspective, is it equality based on rights, happiness, primary goods (i.e., self-respect and freedom of speech), functioning in health? Perhaps the best fit is to suggest that health literacy is an inequality of opportunity in health. Rosa Dias's (2010) definition, based on Roemer's (2002) model, is that, "Equality of opportunity in health attains when average health outcomes are identical across types, at fixed levels of effort." (p. 254). This means that, on average, all those who adopt identical lifestyles should be entitled to experience a similar health status, irrespective of their circumstances. Such a situation corresponds to a full nullification of the effect of circumstances—keeping untouched the differences in health outcomes that are caused solely by effort (Rosa Dias, 2010). As an economic analyst, how does one measure inequality of opportunity in health? Equality can be formulated by gaps, ratios, shortfalls, or ginis (N.B. The gini coefficient is a measure of the inequality of a distribution [e.g., opportunity], a value of 0 expressing total equality and a value of 1 maximal inequality).

Rosa Dias (2009, 2010) used a *gini-opportunity index* and a *conditional equality* approach when applied to a UK longitudinal study. He (2009) found that at least 21% of the health inequalities observed in adulthood were due to inequality of opportunity. An individual's health literacy status appears to be fundamentally mediated through both circumstance (i.e., illegitimate source of inequality) and effort (i.e., legitimate source of inequality). Rosa Dias (2009) concluded: "Since the influence of circumstances on health is often channelled through effort, key complementary policies to reduce health inequalities may need to be implemented outside the health care system and, in particular, in the educational sector." (p. 1073). In the US, Bennett et al. (2009) studied older adults and their health literacy status; they concluded that below basic health literacy contributes to disparities associated with race/ethnicity and educational attainment in self-rated health and with some preventative health behaviours.

As social disparities tend to exist outside of the health care sector, they are considered to be distinct from health inequality or disparity issues. Because of a clustering of risks, those with limited literacy are more likely to be living in a neighbourhood under circumstances that are associated with high rates of chronic disease (Schillinger, 2011). Ratzan's (2001) 21st Century Field Model presents a conceptual framework to link health literacy application of primary, secondary, and tertiary medical prevention with determinants of health (i.e., social, physical, and environmental), education, income, and vulnerability or risk factors. Ratzan concluded that, in order to attain health literacy, policy makers and leaders outside of the health sector must be aware of the critical elements that contribute to health illiteracy. This suggests the importance of supporting general adult education programs in vulnerable communities.

By definition, a public health approach to addressing health literacy would be directed to all of the population and not just those members of the population at the tail of the distribution. This is the prime difference between strategies taking a public health approach and those reflecting a more individualized and often clinical approach. Health Literacy Missouri (HLM) is the *poster boy* of organisations that view health literacy as a public health issue. The start-up costs and the long-term vision of such an approach require political will, ample funding, and determined leadership. How to evaluate HLM's approach to health literacy is open to debate. Few studies are designed to examine all levels of all possible health outcomes.

Parker's health literacy framework (2009) also allows health literacy to be neatly motivated to policy makers—if health literacy is viewed as a health inequalities/disparities issue, it mainly considers the skills/abilities of an individual or of specific groups. Alternatively, if health literacy is seen as a public health issue, policy makers would need to focus on lessening the demands of the health care system for all citizens.

Policy makers are often faced with gaps in the research/knowledge base, leaving policy to be sometimes developed on the basis of so-called good practice (DHE, 2007). Good practice in health literacy may include the widespread use of patient initiatives such as Ask Me 3™ (National Patient Safety Foundation, n.d.) and Speak Up™ (Joint Commission, n.d.), implementation of clear signage in hospitals, or the use of plain-language in the wording of health insurance or other medical documents. Arguably, Volandes, and Paasche-Orlow (2007) best summarized the ethos that any health care system should view health literacy as:

> Instead of assuming literacy and then trying to retrofit care for low literacy patients as some form of speciality service, application of the maximin principle (Rawlsian approach) leads us to the conclusion that the standard of care should be reoriented to the needs of health consumers with limited literacy. (p. 6)

CASE STUDY – ENGLAND

The DHE (2008), under the Labour government, viewed health literacy as a key part of its health inequalities strategy. Although no official documentation has yet been produced, it is likely that the current coalition government will have a different ideological viewpoint on health literacy. As part of the Big Society program (Prime Minister's Office, 2010) that aims "to create a climate that empowers local people and communities" (para. 3), health literacy would fit into the development of the strong communities thread. It is also likely that governmental policy would follow an informed choice rationale that fosters the development of personal and social responsibility (see Chapter 3 for more on informed choice).

Regrettably however, there has been very little research into health literacy in England or the rest of the UK (Protheroe, Nutbeam, and Rowlands, 2009). To date, the most notable academic research has shown that the REALM is a valid screening tool for use in clinical practices (Ibrahim et al., 2008). A systematic review (Easton, Entwistle, and Williams, 2010) and a UK interview study (von Wagner, Knight, Steptoe, and Wardle, 2007) both concluded that limited health literacy is associated with fewer healthy lifestyle behaviours and worse self-rated health.

However, the most exciting health literacy intervention is the Skilled for Health (SfH) program (ContinYou, n.d.; see Chapter 5 for more on SfH). The

Tavistock Institute and Shared Intelligence (2009) conducted a joint evaluation on the second phase of the trial with 1,600 participants in 17 sites. In this pilot study, the array of projects aimed at different population samples (e.g., prison, city council employees, Royal Mail employees) made it virtually impossible to do a traditional cost-benefit or cost-effectiveness economic evaluation. (Cost-benefit analysis [CBA] requires program consequences to be valued in monetary units, thus enabling the analyst to make a direct comparison of a program's incremental cost with its incremental consequences in commensurate units of measurement. Cost-effectiveness analysis [CEA] is a form of full economic evaluation where both the costs and consequences of alternative health programs or treatments are examined with its consequences most often measured in natural health outcome units, such as cost per cases prevented [Drummond, Sculpher, Torrance, O'Brien, and Stoddart, 2005].) The Tavistock report did highlight that the average cost per participant recruited was just over £600.

In this current climate of disinvestment—defined by Elshaug, Hiller, Tunis, and Moss (2007) as the processes of (partially or completely) withdrawing health resources from any existing health care practices, procedures, technologies, or pharmaceuticals that are deemed to deliver little or no health gain for their cost and, thus, not efficient health resource allocations—the economic sustainability and value of an initiative like SfH will receive intense scrutiny. The key question is: Should components of SfH be accessible to everyone through the National Health Service (NHS)? If SfH is not funded through the NHS budget, then the criteria for assessing initiatives lie with the designated budget holder. However, if we consider that SfH affects the health budget then, funding for research into health literacy projects aimed at the whole population will be decided by the National Institute of Health Research (NIHR) Public Health Research (PHR) program as noted by the following statement:

> Evaluation for funding will be based firstly on the submissions of public health importance, and then on its scientific quality, feasibility and value for money. The research findings of projects funded by the NIHR PHR programme will be published for stakeholders to consider. (NIHR PHR, personal communication, February 18, 2010)

Also, it is within the remit of NICE to evaluate public health interventions. NICE (2009) published the process it uses to develop public health guidance that includes a section on incorporating health economics. The issue then for health literacy interventions consistent with public health goals becomes whether the NIHR PHR requirements for economic evaluation would differ from NICE's requirements. Both NIHR PHR and NICE accept invitations regarding potential explorative themes; therefore, it would be reasonable to expect that dialogue with both organisations would clarify what economic analyses should accompany a health literacy proposal.

Accepting that the additional cost of limited health literacy is 3–5% of the total health care cost per year (Eichler et al., 2009), if this figure were applied to the NHS, it would mean that limited health literacy costs the NHS somewhere in the region of £3–5bn annually. More robust evidence using English figures would be a great starting point in raising the awareness of health literacy in the English health care system. At an individual level, there are several longitudinal studies (e.g., National Child Development Study) that would generate interesting data for analysis, should a health literacy component be piggybacked onto the existing survey. Competition for questions on surveys is fierce, and the advocacy community would need to put forth a compelling case for the inclusion of health literacy components.

The Expert Patients Programme for patients with chronic conditions is an example of how effectiveness and cost-effectiveness research has been conducted in England (Kennedy et al., 2007; Richardson et al., 2008). One important consideration for health literacy-themed interventions may well be the need to collect health status utility scores. In health outcomes analyses, utility is a number between 0 and 1 that is assigned to a state of health or an outcome; perfect health has a value of 1, and death has a value of 0. NICE's preferred measure of health-related quality of life (HRQoL) is the EQ-5D (NICE, 2008). EQ-5D is a standardised instrument for use as a measure of health outcome. Applicable to a wide range of health conditions and treatments, it provides a simple descriptive profile and a single index value for health status. Therefore, before and after implementation of the health literacy intervention, the research team may need to collect this data in order to perform an economic evaluation. NICE uses the quality adjusted life year (QALY) as the generic measure of health effects. In health technology appraisals, NICE uses cost-utility analysis (CUA)—a form of evaluation that focuses particular attention on the quality of the health outcome produced or forgone by health programs or treatments (Drummond et al., 2005). Unofficially, a technology (e.g., drug) is deemed to be cost-effective if the cost per QALY is less than £30,000 per QALY. However, criticism of the EQ-5D/QALY methodology is that it does not pick up the subtle yet important changes to patients' health status. This lack of specificity could be problematic for a health literacy-themed intervention because the health outcomes often measured are factors such as improved skills or confidence in dealing with their health condition.

Griffin, Sculpher, and Rice (2010) discussed a potential framework for an economic evaluation of public health interventions. Central to this discussion is whether evaluation should be by CEA or by CBA. For health literacy, the use of compensation tests in public health interventions that span across different government sectors may be important (Claxton, Sculpher, and Culyer, 2007). Therefore, for an initiative such as SfH, the evaluation will need to consider what costs are included and what benefits are measured across the different government sectors (e.g., Department of Education and Department of Health).

The remedy to low health literacy may be skills/education training that may require large up-front costs, and the payoffs may not be that easily measured. In general medical practice, reimbursement is linked to the quality and outcomes framework (QOF; NICE, 2011). Currently, the QOF does not have any indicators to improving health literacy as a specific intervention. General medical practitioners have been shown to respond to incentives (Sutton, Elder, Guthrie, and Watt, 2007). If there were health literacy indicators, then NICE would pilot these new indicators. Note that research on the composition of such indicators would need to be conducted prior to implementation.

The way NHS hospitals operate can be viewed as an extension of the principal–agent model (i.e., DHE and NHS hospital, respectively). In 2001, performance ratings were introduced with each acute hospital receiving a star rating (0–3 stars). One incentive for achieving a three-star rating is financial reward for the hospital. From April 2009, the incremental introduction of patient-related outcome measures came into effect. Linking hospital performance measurement criteria to health literacy may be an avenue worth pursuing.

While it is quite a pedestrian comment to recommend that more health literacy research be conducted, advances in health literacy policy and practice in England are unlikely to proceed without further evidence of its value. There is a need to establish priorities. Should research be focused on gathering more robust prevalence data or on evaluating interventions? What should be borne in mind by the health literacy advocacy community are the processes through which decision-making bodies operate. Understanding the importance of economic analysis to these processes is critical. Presently in England, health literacy operates in a *data desert*; but the potential to assess the degree to which associations between health literacy and medical costs are causal are there. All that is needed is political will and the necessary pounds to support the priorities for health literacy research and evaluation.

CONCLUSION

This chapter used the health literacy framework to give an economic primer in discussing both sides of the *health literacy coin*. A two-pronged attack on improving individuals' skills and reducing complexity in the health care system is recommended. How health literacy is motivated to decision makers and budget holders makes a difference to an economic analyst—be it as a health inequalities or a public health issue. Therefore, the advocacy community needs to be cognizant of these differences. It is imperative that the research community be aware of the economic evidence requirements in promoting health literacy to the various decision makers within the health care system.

Health literacy, just like financial literacy, will have an even greater role to play in future society. Global organizations such as the World Health Organization and the United Nations are embracing the health literacy perspective (Mayagah and Mitic, 2009; United Nations, 2010). The US has a National Action Plan (US Department of Health and Human Services, Office of Disease Prevention and Health Promotion 2010), and more states (e.g., Maryland, New Jersey) are now forming health literacy initiatives/coalitions. On one side of the coin, "Every citizen needs to become a health literate public health practitioner" (Carmona, 2011); but on the other side, it is the responsibility of the health care system to ensure that this goal is achieved in a cost-effective manner.

Questions for Reflection

1) How can health literacy advocates integrate the economic argument into their advocacy efforts?
2) What challenges and opportunities are advocates likely to confront as they engage in this economic discussion with policy makers?

ACKNOWLEDGMENTS

An earlier version of this work was presented at the June 2010 Health Economists Study Group meeting held in Cork, Ireland. The author would like to acknowledge helpful comments and encouragement from the Editors, Dr. Urs Brügger, Prof. Antonio Trujillo, Prof. Ruth Parker, and colleagues at Johns Hopkins School of Public Health, University of York, and Trinity College Dublin.

REFERENCES

Baker, D. W. (2006). The meaning and the measure of health literacy. *Journal of General Internal Medicine, 21*(8), 878-883. doi:10.1111/j.1525-1497.2006.00540.x.

Baker, D. W., Wolf, M. S., Feinglass, J., Thompson, J. A., Gazmararian, J. A., and Huang, J. (2007). Health literacy and mortality among elderly persons. *Archives of Internal Medicine, 167*(14), 1503-1509. doi:<p>10.1001/archinte.167.14.1503</p>.

Bennett, I. M., Chen, J., Soroui, J. S., and White, S. (2009). The contribution of health literacy to disparities in self-rated health status and preventive health behaviors in older adults. *Annals of Family Medicine, 7*(3), 204-211. doi:10.1370/afm.940.

Berkman, N. D., Sheridan, S. L., Donahue, K. E., Halpern, D. J., Viera, A., Crotty, K., ... and Viswanathan, M. (2011, March). *Health literacy interventions and outcomes: An updated systematic review* (Evidence Report/Technology Assessment No. 199; AHRQ Publication Number 11-E006). Rockville, MD: Agency for Healthcare Research and Quality.

Carmona, R. H. (2011, May 31). *The importance of health literacy* (Health Literacy Out Loud #59) [Audio podcast]. Retrieved from http://www.healthliteracyoutloud.com/2011/05/31/health-literacy-out-loud-59-surgeon-general-richard-h-carmona-m-d-m-p-h-facs-talks-about-the-importance-of-health-literacy/#more-190.

Cebul, R. D., Rebitzer, J. B., Taylor, L. J., and Votruba, M. (2008). Organizational fragmentation and care quality in the U.S. healthcare system. *Journal of Economic Perspectives, 22*(4), 93-113. doi:10.1257/jep.22.4.93.

Cho, Y. I., Lee, S. Y., Arozullah, A. M., and Crittenden, K. S. (2008). Effects of health literacy on health status and health service utilization amongst the elderly. *Social Science and Medicine*, *66*(8), 1809-1816. doi:10.1016/j.socscimed.2008.01.003.

Claxton, K., Sculpher, M., and Culyer, A. J. (2007). *Mark versus Luke? Appropriate methods for the evaluation of public health interventions* (CHE Research Paper 31). York, England: University of York Centre for Health Economics. Available from http://econpapers.repec.org/paper/chyrespap/31cherp.htm.

Clement, S., Ibrahim, S., Crichton, N., Wolf, M. S., and Rowlands, G. (2009). Complex interventions to improve the health of people with limited literacy: A systematic review. *Patient Education and Counseling*, *75*(3), 340-351. doi:10.1016/j.pec.2009.01.008.

ContinYou. (n.d.). *What is Skilled for Health?* Retrieved from http://www.continyou.org.uk/health_and_well_being/skilled_health/what_skilled_health.

Department of Health, England. (2007). *Review of the health inequalities infant mortality PSA target*. London, England.: Author. Available from http://www.dh.gov.uk/en/Publicationsandstatistics/Publications/PublicationsPolicyAndGuidance/DH_065544.

Department of Health, England. (2008). *Health inequalities: Progress and next steps*. London, England: Author. Available from http://www.dh.gov.uk/en/Publicationsandstatistics/Publications/PublicationsPolicyAndGuidance/DH_085307.

DeWalt, D. A., Malone, R. M., Bryant, M. E., Kosnar, M. C., Corr, K. E., Rothman, R. L., and Pignone, M. P. (2006). A heart failure self-management program for patients of all literacy levels: A randomized, controlled trial. *BMC Health Services Research*, *6*, 30. doi:10.1186/1472-6963-6-30.

Drummond, M., Sculpher, M., Torrance, G., O'Brien, B., and Stoddart, G. (2005). *Methods for the economic evaluation of health care programmes* (3rd ed.). London, England: Oxford University Press.

Easton, P., Entwistle, V. A., and Williams, B. (2010). Health in the "hidden population" of people with low literacy: A systematic review of the literature. *BMC Public Health*, *10*, 459. doi:10.1186/1471-2458-10-459.

Eichler, K., Wieser, S., and Brügger, U. (2009). The costs of limited health literacy: A systematic review. *International Journal of Public Health*, *54*(5), 313-324. doi:10.1007/s00038-009-0058-2.

Elshaug, A., Hiller, J., Tunis, S., and Moss, J. (2007). Challenges in Australian policy processes for disinvestment from existing, ineffective health care practices. *Australia and New Zealand Health Policy*, *4*(1), 23. doi:10.1186/1743-8462-4-23.

European Commission. (2007). *Together for health: A strategic approach for the EU 2008-2013* [White paper]. Brussels, Belgium: Author. Available from http://europa.eu/legislation_summaries/public_health/european _health_strategy/c11579_en.htm.

Friedland, R. (1998, October). New estimates of the high costs of inadequate health literacy. In *Proceedings of Pfizer Conference "Promoting Health Literacy: A Call to Action"* (pp. 6-10). Washington, DC: Pfizer Inc.

Fuchs, V. (1974/1998). *Who shall live? Health, economics and social choice* (3rd ed.). New York, NY: Basic Books.

Griffin, S., Sculpher, M., and Rice, N. (2010). Use of economic methods to evaluate the cost effectiveness of public health interventions. In A. Killoran and M. P. Kelly (Eds.), *Evidence-based public health: Effectiveness and efficiency* (pp. 110-127). Oxford, England: Oxford University Press.

Grossman, M. (1972). On the concept of health capital and the demand for health. *Journal of Political Economy*, *80*(2), 223-255.

Hasnain-Wynia, R., and Wolf, M. S. (2010). Promoting health care equity: Is health literacy a missing link? *Health Services Research*, *45*(4), 897-903. doi:10.1111/j.1475-6773.2010.01134.x.

Health Literacy Iowa. (n.d.). *Low health literacy costs Iowans more than $2 billion each year* [Online news release]. Retrieved from http://www.ihs.org/body.cfm?id=459.

Howard, D. H., Gazmararian, J., and Parker, R. M. (2005). The impact of low health literacy on the medical costs of Medicare managed care enrollees. *American Journal of Medicine*, *118*(4), 371-377. doi:10.1016/j.amjmed.2005.01.010.

Howard-Pitney, B., Winkleby, M. A., Albright, C. L., Bruce, B., and Fortmann, S. P. (1997). The Stanford nutrition action program: A dietary fat intervention for low-literacy adults. *American Journal of Public Health*, *87*(12), 1971-1976.

Hutton, J., McGrath, C., Frybourg, J.-M., Tremblay, M., Bramley-Harker, E., and Henshall, C. (2006). Framework for describing and classifying decision-making systems using technology assessment to determine the reimbursement of health technologies (fourth hurdle systems).

International Journal of Technology Assessment in Health Care, *22*(1), 10-18.

Ibrahim, S. Y., Reid, F., Shaw, A., Rowlands, G., Gomez, G. B., Chesnokov, M., and Ussher, M. (2008). Validation of a health literacy screening tool (REALM) in a UK population with coronary heart disease. *Journal of Public Health*, *30*(4), 449-455. doi:10.1093/pubmed/fdn059.

Joint Commission. (n.d.). *Speak-up™ homepage.* Retrieved from http://www.jointcommission.org/speakup.aspx.

Kenkel, D. S. (1994). The demand for preventative medical care. *Applied Economics*, *26*(4), 313-25.

Kennedy, A., Reeves, D., Bower, P., Lee, V., Middleton, E., Richardson, G., ... Rogers, A. (2007). The effectiveness and cost effectiveness of a national lay-led self care support programme for patients with long-term conditions: A pragmatic randomised controlled trial. *Journal of Epidemiology and Community Health*, *61*(3), 254-261. doi:10.1136/jech.2006.053538.

Kirsch, I. S., Roter, D., Pisano, S., and King, A. (2010, October). *Health literacy: Measuring the other side of the coin.* Invited panel presentation to the Annual Research Conference on Health Literacy, Bethesda, MD.

Mayagah, K., and Mitic, W. (2009, October). *Health literacy and health promotion: Definitions, concepts and examples in the eastern Mediterranean region.* Working discussion document presented at the WHO 7th Global Conference on Health Promotion "Promoting Health and Development: Closing the Implementation Gap," Nairobi, Kenya. Available from http://www.who.int/healthpromotion/conferences/7gchp/documents/en/.

McCormack, L. (2009). What is health literacy and how do we measure it? In *Proceedings of the Institute of Medicine Workshop "Measures of Health Literacy,"* (pp. 29-34). Washington DC: The National Academies Press. Available from http://www.nap.edu/openbook.php?record_id=12690 andpage=R1.

National Institute for Health and Clinical Excellence. (2008). *Guide to the methods of technology appraisal.* Retrieved from http://www.nice.org.uk/aboutnice/howwework/devnicetech/technologyappraisalprocessguides/guidetothemethodsoftechnologyappraisal.jsp.

National Institute for Health and Clinical Excellence. (2009). *Developing NICE public health guidance.* Retrieved from http://www.nice.org.uk/aboutnice/howwework/developingnicepublichealthguidance/developing_nice_public_health_guidance.jsp.

National Institute for Health and Clinical Excellence. (2011). *About the quality and outcomes framework (QOF)*. Retrieved from http://www.nice.org.uk/aboutnice/qof/qof.jsp.

National Patient Safety Foundation. (n.d.). *Homepage*. Retrieved from http://www.npsf.org/askme3/.

Osborn, C. Y., Paasche-Orlow, M. K., Bailey, S. C., and Wolf, M. S. (2011). The mechanisms linking health literacy to behavior and health status. *American Journal of Health Behavior, 35*(1), 118-128.

Osborn, C. Y., Paasche-Orlow, M. K., Davis, T. C., and Wolf, M. S. (2007). Health literacy: An overlooked factor in understanding HIV health disparities. *American Journal of Preventive Medicine, 33*(5), 374-378. doi:10.1016/j.amepre.2007.07.022.

Paasche-Orlow, M. K., and Wolf, M. S. (2007). The causal pathways linking health literacy to health outcomes. *American Journal of Health Behavior, 31*(S1), S19-26. doi:10.5555/ajhb.2007.31.supp.S19.

Paasche-Orlow, M. K., and Wolf, M. S. (2010). Promoting health literacy research to reduce health disparities. *Journal of Health Communication, 15*(S2), S34-41. doi:10.1080/10810730.2010.499994.

Parker, R. M. (2009). Measuring health literacy: What? So what? Now what? In *Proceedings of the Institute of Medicine Workshop "Measures of Health Literacy,"* (pp. 91-98). Washington DC: The National Academies Press. Available from http://www.nap.edu/openbook.php?record_id=12690andpage=R1.

Pleasant, A. (2009). Health literacy measurement: A brief review and proposal. In *Proceedings of the Institute of Medicine Workshop "Measures of Health Literacy,"* (pp. 17-22). Washington DC: The National Academies Press. Available from http://www.nap.edu/openbook.php?record_id=12690andpage=R1.

Pleasant, A., and Kuruvilla, S. (2008). A tale of two health literacies: Public health and clinical approaches to health literacy. *Health Promotion International, 23*(2), 152-159. doi:10.1093/heapro/dan001.

Prime Minister's Office. (2010, May). *Government launches Big Society programme*. London, England: Author. Retrieved from http://www.number10.gov.uk/news/big-society/.

Protheroe, J., Nutbeam, D., and Rowlands, G. (2009). Health literacy: A necessity for increasing participation in health care. *British Journal of General Practice, 59*(567), 721-723. doi:10.3399/bjgp09X472584.

Ratzan, S. C. (2001). Health literacy: Communication for the public good. *Health Promotion International, 16*(2), 207-214.

Ratzan, S. C, and Parker, R. M. (2000). Introduction. In *National library of medicine current bibliographies in medicine: Health literacy* (NLM Pub. No. CBM 2000-1); C. R. Sedlen, M. Zorn, S. C. Ratzan, and N. Lurie (Eds.). Bethesda, MD: National Institutes of Health, US Department of Health and Human Services.

Richardson, G., Kennedy, A., Reeves, D., Bower, P., Lee, V., Middleton, E., ... Rogert, A. (2008). Cost effectiveness of the Expert Patients Programme (EPP) for patients with chronic conditions. *Journal of Epidemiology and Community Health, 62*(4), 361-367. doi:10.1136/jech.2006.057430.

Roemer, J. (2002). Equality of opportunity: A progress report. *Social Choice and Welfare, 19*(2), 455-471.

Rosa Dias, P. (2009). Inequality of opportunity in health: Evidence from a UK cohort study. *Health Economics, 18*(9), 1057-1074. doi:10.1002/hec.1535.

Rosa Dias, P. (2010). Modelling opportunity in health under partial observability of circumstances. *Health Economics, 19*(3), 252-264. doi:10.1002/hec.1584.

Sanders, L. M., Thompson, V. T., and Wilkinson, J. D. (2007). Caregiver health literacy and the use of child health services. *Pediatrics, 119*(1), e86-92. doi:10.1542/peds.2005-1738.

Schillinger, D. (2011). Will improving health literacy reduce health disparities for vulnerable populations? In *Proceedings of the Institute of Medicine Workshop "Innovations in Health Literacy,"* (pp. 12-18). Washington DC: The National Academies Press. Available from http://www.nap.edu/catalog.php?record_id=13016.

Scott, T. L., Gazmararian, J. A., Williams, M. V., and Baker, D. W. (2002). Health literacy and preventive health care use among Medicare enrollees in a managed care organization. *Medical Care, 40*(5), 395-404.

Smith, S. K., Trevena, L., Simpson, J. M., Barratt, A., Nutbeam, D., and McCaffery, K. J. (2010). A decision aid to support informed choices about bowel cancer screening among adults with low education: Randomised controlled trial. *BMJ (Clinical Research Ed.), 341*, c5370.

Spycher, S. (2006). *Okonomische Aspekte der Gesundheitskompetenz* [Economic aspects of health literacy]. Berne, Switzerland: BASS [Buro fur Arbeits und Sozialpolitische Studien].

Stinnett, A. A., and Mullahy, J. (1998). Net health benefits: A new framework for the analysis of uncertainty in cost-effectiveness analysis. *Medical Decision Making, 18*(S2), S68-80.

Sutton, M., Elder, R., Guthrie, B., and Watt, G. (2007). *What quality improvement did the Quality and Outcomes Framework produce?* Paper presented at the Health Economists Study Group, Aberdeen, Scotland.

Tavistock Institute and Shared Intelligence. (2009). *Evaluation of the second phase of the Skilled for Health Programme: Final evaluation report.* London, England: Authors.

United Nations. (2010). Health literacy and the Millennium Development Goals: United Nations Economic and the Social Council (ECOSOC) regional meeting background paper (abstracted). *Journal of Health Communication, 15*(S2), S211-223. doi:10.10810730.2010.499996.

United States Department of Health and Human Services, Office of Disease Prevention and Health Promotion. (2010). *National action plan to improve health literacy.* Washington, DC: Author.

van Servellen, G., Nyamathi, A., Carpio, F., Pearce, D., Garcia-Teague, L., Herrera, G., and Lombardi, E. (2005). Effects of a treatment adherence enhancement program on health literacy, patient-provider relationships, and adherence to HAART among low-income HIV-positive Spanish-speaking Latinos. *AIDS Patient Care and STDs, 19*(11), 745-759. doi:10.1089/apc.2005.19.745.

Vernon, J. A. (2009). *Health policy brief: The high economic cost of low health literacy in Wisconsin.* Retrieved from http://www4.uwm.edu/publichealth/onpublichealth/upload/ Kanack-Handout Article.pdf.

Vernon, J. A., Trujilo, A., and Keener Hughen, W. (2007). *Health policy brief: The high economic cost of low health literacy in Missouri.* Retrieved from http://www.healthliteracymissouri.org/uploads/HLM/pdfs/Vernon_Report. pdf.

Vernon, J. A., Trujillo, A., Rosenbaum, S., and DeBuono, B. (2007). *Low health literacy: Implications for national health policy.* Retrieved from http://www.gwumc.edu/sphhs/ departments/healthpolicy/dhp_publications/pub_uploads/dhpPublication_ 3AC9A1C2-5056-9D20-3D4BC6786DD46 B1B.pdf.

Volandes, A. E., and Paasche-Orlow, M. K. (2007). Health literacy, health inequality and a just healthcare system. *American Journal of Bioethics, 7*(11), 5-10. doi:10.1080/15265160701638520.

von Wagner, C., Knight, K., Steptoe, A., and Wardle, J. (2007). Functional health literacy and health-promoting behaviour in a national sample of British adults. *Journal of Epidemiology and Community Health, 61*(12), 1086-1090. doi:10.1136/jech.2006.053967.

Weider Ocampo, B. (2009). Developing and testing a CAPHS® health literacy item set. In *Proceedings of the Institute of Medicine Workshop "Measures of Health Literacy,"* (pp. 81-84). Washington DC: The National Academies Press. Available from http://www.nap.edu/openbook.php? record_id=12690andpage=R1.

Weiss, B. D., and Palmer, R. (2004). Relationship between health care costs and very low literacy skills in a medically needy and indigent Medicaid population. *Journal of the American Board of Family Practice, 17*(1), 44-47.

Wieser, S., Moschetti, K., Eichler, K., Holly, A., and Brügger, U. (2008). *Health literacy - An economic perspective and data for Switzerland; Part 2: A review of health literacy measures and a cost assessment of limited health literacy.* Winterhur and Lausanne, Switzerland: Winterhur Institute of Health Economics. Retrieved from http://www.gesundheitsfoerderung. ch/pdf_doc_xls/e/GFPstaerken/Health-Literacy-Part-2.pdf.

Wolf, M. S., Gazmararian, J. A., and Baker, D. W. (2007). Health literacy and health risk behaviors among older adults. *American Journal of Preventive Medicine, 32*(1), 19-24. doi:10.1016/j.amepre.2006.08.024.

In: Health Literacy in Context   ISBN: 978-1-61942-921-5
Eds.: D.Begoray, D.Gillis, G.Rowlands © 2012 Nova Science Publishers, Inc.

Chapter 8

CONCLUDING THOUGHTS AND THE FUTURE OF HEALTH LITERACY

Deborah L. Begoray[*], Gillian Rowlands and Doris E. Gillis

ABSTRACT

In this concluding chapter, the Editors reflect on the unique opportunity presented by the sharing of interdisciplinary and international experiences and perspectives in the complex and important area of health literacy. We identify some key themes that flow through the chapters in the book, including the definitions and conceptions of health literacy and its measurement, issues of power, the impact of policy, and concern for health inequalities. Finally, we offer some conjectures about the future of health literacy and final questions for reflection for readers.

INTRODUCTION

Health Literacy in Context: International Perspectives is a volume of multiplicities: multiple authors, topics, countries, and perspectives. The authors are doctors, nurses, nutritionists, pharmacists, psychologists, educators, social workers, administrators, economists, researchers, and

---

[*] Corresponding author: E-mail: dbegoray@uvic.ca.

professors. Many wear more than one hat within the health literacy spectrum of multiple interests, perhaps as a health promotion specialist and university professor or as a primary care physician and head of a health literacy network. They also deal with different populations both in terms of age (e.g., children, adolescents, adults, seniors) and across ethnic diversities as people move and migrate to different countries, bringing their health traditions with them. The topics chosen for the chapters, however, we see as common concerns for those currently engaging with the multifaceted concept of health literacy: definitions and measurement, healthy lifestyles, health outcomes, lifelong learning, community-based interventions, and the economic implications of low health literacy and of developing health-literate citizens, systems, and communities. While the perspectives are many, the topics are universal. We suggest the union of perspectives with topics provides a strong set of ideas for those interested in the evolving field of health literacy. The multidisciplinary nature of the original 2010 conference has evolved into interdisciplinary collaborations as authors have worked together to prepare their chapters.

As we edited this book and reviewed its content at length, we have been reminded of the very contextual nature of health literacy. This fact seems to arise, at least in part, from the widely varying nature of health systems across the countries represented. Authors have made the point that, even within their countries, local regions often have unique systems and practice settings resulting in heterogeneous health policy and practice guidelines. Notably, the same heterogeneity characterizes other systems (e.g., education, adult literacy, social services), which also has implications for health literacy. Authors have highlighted and demonstrated, through examples from the field, the close ties between health literacy and the cultural context that determine how people access, understand, evaluate, communicate, and decide whether or not to use information for their health. Given the multicultural make-up of many communities, appreciation of this cultural diversity comes to the foreground when looking at applications of health literacy in order to build capacity for achieving positive health outcomes.

Different countries provide more or less leadership and financial resources to assist the harmonious union of users and services needed to ensure that health literacy is a shared responsibility between users and providers within health systems. As pointed out by several authors, health literacy is situated in a broader policy context, largely influenced by the ideology and priorities of governing bodies that frame policy for health and education. As we complete this volume, the Western world has moved into challenging economic times that are having an unprecedented impact on health and education funding in many jurisdictions. Uncertain times create obstacles to, as well as opportunities for, innovative ideas and interventions. As an emerging concept and evolving field of practice, health literacy will no doubt be shaped by these new economic realities.

Therefore, health literacy seems, within the topics and through the perspectives pursued in this book, to be at a crucial crossroad. Research shows that a higher level of health literacy is correlated with a number of positive health outcomes and that health literacy can contribute to the amelioration of health costs. Nevertheless, the growth of a more health-literate population calls for a variety of professionals and citizens—teachers and students, policy makers and social activists, researchers and practitioners—working with individuals and groups within their varied contexts. It is within these largely unique situations that health literacy will find its place and continue to evolve in concept as it becomes embedded in the way we practice.

At this point then, it seems important to remind readers of the context within which this volume was engendered (for an overview of other key events in the history of health literacy, see Chapter 1 *Introduction*). In 2007, the Department of Health in England, recognizing the importance of health literacy to patients, citizens, and the National Health Service, funded the initiation of the Health Literacy Group UK. One aim of the Group was, and is, to build the health literacy evidence base in the United Kingdom (UK). The Group recognized the extensive research undertaken by colleagues from other countries; it wished to review this evidence and, where appropriate, adapt and build on this work to improve health and health services. As one way to accomplish this task, an international conference was organized and held in February 2010 at London South Bank University—a university well suited to host this meeting given its multicultural population and setting in the heart of London. The conference presentations by this book's authors formed the basis of *Health Literacy in Context: International Perspectives.*

In this final chapter, we address the various themes that wove the presentations (now chapters) together and provided unifying elements to the multiple perspectives described above. These themes include the definitions and conceptions of health literacy and its measurement, issues of power, the impact of policy, and concern for health inequalities. Finally, we offer some thoughts about the future of health literacy; that is, where we believe the field might move in the future.

THEMES

Theme 1: Definitions Influence Health Literacy Approaches and Measurement

What is health literacy really? The answers are multiple but astute readers will see that the definitions and conceptions revolve around the idea of people's ability to interact successfully with health information. As Rudd, McCray, and Nutbeam lay out the conceptual issues in Chapter 2 *Health Literacy and Definitions of Terms*, they describe the defining of health literacy as problematic and a source of much debate among contributors to this growing field of study and practice. It is not surprising that the authors of each succeeding chapter provide readers with their choice of definition and understanding of health literacy from the literature. Their choices reflect the conceptions most appropriate to issues within their particular area(s) of expertise and relevant to the broader policy context of their respective country and location. At first sight, readers might be forgiven for assuming that the multiplicity of concepts and definitions is a disadvantage; the argument might be that multiple definitions of a concept such as health literacy, no matter how clear each is, bring potential for confusion. Moreover, how can we move ahead as a field of practice without a common understanding of health literacy? As the authors of each chapter demonstrate, however, the breadth of health literacy topics and perspectives—and the multiple ways in which interventions can impact people and their lives—could not be captured in one definition. The variety of concepts and definitions discussed throughout the book enables the complex construct of health literacy to be viewed and explored using different paradigms and within different contexts. Within the settings of schoolrooms and hospitals, doctors' offices and community health centres, pharmacies and food stores, the idea of a *best* definition varies—and so it should. Readers might examine chapters for the definition they find most suitable to their context and consider why they prefer one over the other.

In our view, this freedom to choose and defend one's choice of definition is essential now and as the field of health literacy expands; indeed, we speculate that the present concepts and definitions will evolve as the field develops and identifies even more areas where health literacy is applicable and relevant to practice. We encourage readers—students, professors, researchers, activists, and practitioners—to be aware of the varying definitions of health literacy and to identify those that most closely match their aims, to clarify the definition they use in their work, to examine underlying assumptions, and to contribute new understandings in the future drawn from their research and reflective practice. Ongoing dialogue among scholars and practitioners about the multiple facets of health literacy will help build the theory needed to further define and strengthen the field of health literacy.

The richness and complexity of varying definitions within the field of health literacy is both exciting and challenging for those engaged in research and practice development. While definitions proscribe health literacy, they are also inexplicably connected with the measurement of health literacy abilities. Given its evolving conceptualization and the many contexts in which health literacy is applied, it is not surprising that much remains to be done to develop rigorous means of measurement. As it stands, the health literacy measures that are adopted arise from the definition chosen; and the definition, by nature, influences one's view of health literacy. What measure is wanted? The skill of reading pill bottle labels or the ability to build a website to mobilize a community to seek better health care service access from its government? The skill of explaining to an emotional patient which steps are needed to manage a long-term illness or the ability to evaluate the latest media lifestyle advertisements? Measures will be more or less appropriate to each situation and goal. Some contexts may want or need extensive quantitative measures, while others may call for narratives and themes of qualitative evaluations—or even both.

However challenging measurement might be, without rigorous measurement methods and appropriate tools, it becomes impossible to evaluate interventions, report on progress, argue for funding, or gain the ear of various stakeholders. Readers will see that the authors have used and cited various measures of health literacy. Historically, these have mostly focused on the *functional* or *basic* end of the skills spectrum as being somewhat more straightforward to measure and more useful in clinical contexts (e.g., answering questions such as: Can my patient read this set of instructions?). In their discussion of health literacy and health outcomes in Chapter 4 *Health Literacy and Health Outcomes*, Protheroe, Wolf, and Lee claim that measures used in clinical contexts based on a functional approach to literacy are limited and need to incorporate a broader range of skills and capacities. Currently, more complex instruments in both clinical and general health decision-making contexts are called for as we strive to evaluate critical thinking skills and health attitudes; for example, can this person judge the worth of this health information and is s/he willing, or able, to engage in a recommended activity given the socioeconomic constraints of everyday life? Certainly, as Coughlan discusses in Chapter 7 *Health Literacy: An Economic Perspective*, the general economic impact of health literacy should have a strong influence on government policy. Such policies should recognise the important mediating effects of culture and community as outlined by Levin-Zamir and Wills in Chapter 6 *Health Literacy, Culture, and Community*. In Chapter 2, Rudd, McCray, and Nutbeam argue that more work is especially needed on defining and measuring health literacy in ways that capture the engagement and skills of those in public health and in health care who influence what and how health information is provided within diverse physical and social contexts of health-related activities demanding health literacy skills.

As the field of health literacy continues to expand, we will need measures that capture the wider range of skills inherent in more complex concepts, are sensitive to change, and enable us to make comparisons across contexts. We speculate that this might best be achieved through dialogue between those investigating health literacy from different, albeit complementary, starting points. These interdisciplinary conversations are evident in many of the teams that authored the chapters in this book. Chapter 5 *Health Literacy and Lifelong Learning*, for example, features an educator, a psychologist, a social worker, and a primary care physician—now all university academics—as its authors.

Last but not least, the voices of individuals trying to engage with health information in their various roles as patients, caregivers, consumers, or citizens also have an important place in future conversations about the meaning of health literacy and how health literacy interventions are to be designed, implemented, and evaluated.

Theme 2: Power and Power Shifts Are Features of Health Literacy Contexts

In clinical settings, practitioners and patients undertake a one-to-one relationship in a medical clinic, office, or hospital—settings that are outside peoples' everyday lives (e.g., see Protheroe, Wolf, and Lee in Chapter 4). In these clinical interactions, complex health advice is largely transmitted from the practitioner to the patient, with compliance by the patient being the foremost goal. Historically, the focus for health literacy research in this setting has been an investigation of the mismatch between the literacy and numeracy skills of patients receiving health information and the professional experts transmitting health information, with particular attention being paid to the skills (or lack of skills) of the information recipients. Nutbeam (2009) explored how patients' level of functional health literacy skills can best and most quickly be ascertained and how health services and health information can be better designed to ameliorate the impact of low skills in individual patients. The focus of power in this context has traditionally rested with the practitioners and the health service within which they operate; they have held the information on health, and the responsibility of patients has been to act on the information they are given.

A health promotion approach to health literacy takes a different perspective more in keeping with public health issues and practices. In Chapter 3 *Health Literacy and Healthy Lifestyle Choices*, Gillis and Gray highlight the importance of individuals' lifestyle decisions on promoting health and the inherent tension around the ideological and political issue of individual versus social responsibility for health. This approach shifts the health literacy focus beyond the match, or mismatch, of skills within the practitioner–patient consultation to address the skills that all individuals employ to evaluate health information within the context of their daily lives. Individuals—not just as patients but as consumers, caregivers, and citizens—engage with information about healthy lifestyle behaviours on a daily basis in a variety of contexts beyond health care settings, for example, in the marketplace, through multimedia channels, with family and friends. All individuals should have access to health-promoting information that is relevant and provided in ways that enables them to gain control over their own health. One's sense of autonomy and ability to make and decide whether or not to act on an informed choice is central to the idea of empowerment captured in the notion of health promotion and the World Health Organization's definition of health literacy (1998). This perspective emphasizes the importance of situating health literacy within the context of the broader social determinants of health. As such, it calls for policy that ensures societal factors promote equity of access and opportunity to all citizens so they can engage with information to achieve positive health outcomes. While many governments today tend to place greater responsibility on their citizens to access, understand, and use information to improve their lifestyle, thereby reducing the financial burden of chronic disease, they must ensure that their citizens live in social, economic, and physical environments that allow them to act on this information.

A further shift in power and responsibility occurs when the focus moves from individual health literacy skills to community health literacy skills. In Chapter 6, Levin-Zamir and Wills discuss how supporting communities helps citizens to exert more control over their environment and the social determinants that shape their lives as well as use the collective health resources of the wider community more effectively and efficiently. In the 2010 conference that was the genesis of this book, representatives from several such community groups gave their views on this very issue. Many had become engaged in health literacy as a way of addressing particular local needs, and the projects that were developed had a focus on empowering individuals and communities. A common theme of these presentations was that approaches to working with communities had shifted: no longer did the practitioner hold the power of information dissemination; instead, community groups took an active role by choosing and inviting local specialists to share their expertise as part of a community-led, problem-solving process. Agencies serving sophisticated, health-literate communities may have to adjust to a very different relationship with the people they serve, providing the information required by communities on issues, in settings, and at times that suit the community. In turn, however, agencies and practitioners may find that they have gained valuable allies in the quest for better health care services and programs when trying to leverage government funding to support community-led health interventions.

Ongoing learning and education can support citizen empowerment for better health. As seen in Chapter 5, Begoray, Marshall, Shone, and Rowlands discuss how the education system can support health literacy development throughout the life course and within a variety of settings. Children, adolescents, and younger and older adults need both formal and informal ways to learn about health. Such learning can be provided through education programs within schools and other institutions; increasingly, it is available through community centres, libraries, and in other public venues. *Skilled for Health*, described in Chapter 5, provides an especially important example of how health literacy capacity can be enhanced in the adult population as part of lifelong learning.

Theme 3: Health Literacy Addresses Health Inequalities

Another theme that is featured throughout this volume, and closely tied to the previous theme of power, is the role of health literacy in addressing health inequalities. Health inequalities arising from remediable social and economic causes are well recognized (Commission on the Social Determinants of Health, 2008). Despite efforts to reduce such disparities, the health gap has remained both persistent and resistant to change. Within the health literacy debate, strategies to address health disparities will differ depending on whether a clinical/biomedical or a public health/health promotion approach is adopted.

As described by Protheroe, Wolf, and Lee in Chapter 4, people with low functional health literacy skills face tremendous hurdles in becoming and staying healthy. Within clinical settings, low functional health literacy skills, exacerbated by the devastating impact of poverty and social exclusion, have a real and negative impact on health. They suggest this problem arises in large part through dysfunctional practitioner–patient communication; patients with lower skills are unable to assimilate and act upon the information they are given in the consultation.

A public health approach to health literacy, as described by Gillis and Gray in Chapter 3, takes a different perspective. This approach highlights the importance of lifestyle decisions on promoting health rather than just addressing the management of illness. This approach shifts the focus and point of maximum effective intervention away from the clinical consultation toward the provision of high-quality, readily accessible, health-promoting information to intended populations and the development of their capacity to evaluate and act upon this information within the context of current life events and throughout their life-course. By extending the concept of health literacy from a focus on individual responsibility for personal health management to consider how the social determinants of health—such as limited income, literacy, and social support—often constrain individuals' ability to act on information provided, we acknowledge the relevance of health literacy in addressing health disparities.

The debate on effective approaches to achieve health equality starts with the public (as described above under Theme 2), which needs high-quality, accurate information on these differing approaches. An individualistic approach, exemplified by the clinical/biomedical identification of individual risk combined with strategies to improve communication, is likely to be faster and cheaper to implement. Those who are changing and improving practice guidelines are clinicians and managers employed within the health service; federal or national standards and targets could be designed and applied throughout systems of delivery. If interventions could be tailored to reach marginalized groups and meet the health literacy needs and contexts of those with existing health conditions, reducing inequality of access and of disease control should be relatively easy to measure and demonstrate.

An alternative is a public health/health promotion approach, with co-ordination of health promotion and lifelong learning activities. In Chapter 5, Begoray, Marshall, Shone, and Rowlands describe the importance of the development of health literacy skills at every stage in education—from schools through to adult education. This requires educators, health professionals, and health promotion experts to develop, design, implement, and evaluate interventions that enable the public to learn how to learn about health. The focus of development is not only on knowledge acquisition—modern medicine and health knowledge changes rapidly and information quickly becomes obsolete—but on ways of identifying and evaluating credible sources of information. It involves not only developing an understanding of how lifestyle and the physical and social environment have an impact on health but also providing the skills and resources to take control of adverse circumstances. Such approaches are likely to work best through parallel support of community initiatives and development. The collective skills of communities will be greater than the sum of the individuals within it, and such an approach may reduce inequalities by empowering individuals and communities currently marginalised and at higher risk of developing long-term conditions. The ultimate proof would be that all population groups would have the capacity to effectively manage and assume more control over their own health and that of their communities.

We argue, therefore, for further national debates on the place of health literacy with respect to health inequality issues and the social economic determinants of health, with informed decision-making on the approaches chosen and the outcomes to be realised. Only in this way will all segments of the public realize the increase in positive health outcomes that can be achieved through developing health-literate systems and society.

Theme 4: Policy Has an Important Impact on the Development of Health Literacy

Health literacy capacity does not develop in a vacuum. Citizens, communities, and health practitioners, in partnership with educators, will only be able to develop the health literacy skills they need to improve and maintain health if the social and cultural environment is conducive to such practice. The extent to which a population becomes health literate and able to meet society's increasing demands for health literacy skills, such as those required to navigate through complex health care systems or make healthy choices in the marketplace, is largely dependent on the policies of governments and their political aims.

Internationally, health literacy policy develops within the political philosophies of the day and the wider sweeps of cultural habits and beliefs. In some health care systems, access to health services often requires reading and writing ability, for example, in the US where health care follows the submission of lengthy forms required by health insurers. Health care varies by the insurance that can be afforded by the user. In other more socialized systems, such as those in Canada and the European Union (EU), all citizens can access more or less the same level of care by oral request at a hospital or clinic, although health literacy still has a significant impact on the information and care received. Stableford and Mettger (2007) suggested that health literacy came late in capturing the interest of researchers and policy makers in Canada and Europe because citizens there, in comparison to those in the US, could more easily access health care and information through their nationalized systems and faced fewer navigation issues.

For most Western governments, one of the major reasons for the importance of health literacy at a national policy level is to help address the economic cost of illness, particularly managing the long-term conditions of an aging society and the ever-increasing variety and cost of medical technology and treatment options. In the UK, the Wanless report (2002) highlighted the need to reduce demand for, as well as improve productivity and supply of, health services if health care costs were to be controlled. We believe the approach to reducing healthliteracyrelated issues needs to be led by politicians, acting on the mandate given by their electorate, with policy designed to clearly outline the approach taken and hence the expected outcomes. An important aspect for politicians is that the improvements brought through greater health literacy should ideally be demonstrable within an election cycle. The disadvantage of such short-term approaches is that they may do little to address the underlying causes of low health literacy but may simply ameliorate its worst effects. In contrast, public health, education, and health promotion approaches tend to take much longer to bring about positive change, are potentially more expensive, and are usually more difficult to evaluate. Policy, however, should build capacity for evidence-based practice and minimize costs through enabling the sharing of complementary skills and resources from health and education. The potential benefits of public health approaches enacted in policy are huge: an informed and empowered citizenry in control of its own health.

In many parts of the world, there is a need for a national debate on these issues, followed by informed policy and measurable outcomes tailored to the approach adopted, and with implementation fostered by strong leaders. Only in this way will citizens experience the increase in health that can be brought through developing health-literate systems in society.

THE FUTURE OF HEALTH LITERACY:
WHERE IS THE FIELD GOING?

As we, the Editors, look into the future, it seems to us that the only constant will be change. There can be no doubt that health literacy presently has considerable momentum. A number of future trends seem likely, and we discuss them briefly below.

Continuing Discussion on Definitions and Appropriate Measures

Health literacy will continue to adopt and adapt different definitions and conceptual frameworks. While some will bemoan the lack of agreement in the field, others will applaud its many-faceted nature. Although there is no universally shared definition of health literacy (as this book demonstrates), definitions of health literacy reflecting national perspectives (e.g., in the US, Canada, Wales, Scotland, and Ireland) are emerging; and more activities to establish baseline health literacy levels are being undertaken. More population-based surveys and measures based on specific definitions of health literacy suggest an increasing recognition of the relevance of a more health-literate population. In the EU, an extensive health literacy survey (European Health Literacy Survey, 2011) involving eight countries (i.e., The Netherlands, Greece, Ireland, Austria, Poland, Bulgaria, Germany, Spain) is preparing to release its data as we complete the preparation of this book.

Some researchers, practitioners, and policy makers will no doubt remain faithful to health literacy definitions that are associated with influential groups, such as that of the US Institute of Medicine: "... the degree to which individuals have the capacity to obtain, process, and understand basic health information and services needed to make appropriate health decisions" (Ratzan and Parker, 2000, as cited in Nielsen-Bohlman, Panzer, and Kindig, 2004, p. 20).

Other definitions might be considered more emergent, such as the one commonly used in Canada: "The ability to access, understand, evaluate and communicate information as a way to promote, maintain and improve health in a variety of settings across the life course" (Rootman and Gordon-El-Bihbety, 2008, p. 11). Canada's definition arose from the Expert Panel's engagement with research as reported in the literature and through consultation with practitioners in health and education and with adult learners across the country. Other countries and disciplines will continue to look at expanding the definition of health literacy. Some may add elements of complexity and inclusivity that suit their health promotion and social reconstruction aspirations, while others may prefer to limit the definition to make discrete skills easier to quantify in specific settings and situations.

Power Issues

Influential stakeholders defining the agenda within the field of health literacy, we suggest, will continue to change; and there will be more voice for citizens and community groups, which many might applaud. In addition, however, there will be struggles over how far control of health information and advice should swing away from highly educated medical specialists toward a proliferation of self-proclaimed experts whose views on health may be at best highly eccentric and at worst highly dangerous, with a wide middle ground of largely baseless opinion that may turn out to be good or bad. In this newly open space of health opinion, critical thinking will be even more important as people grapple with controversies such as those surrounding some recent vaccination campaigns or food labelling policies. Community groups, we believe, will enjoy more influence on the ways that health practitioners share their knowledge and expertise.

Growing Importance of Technology

Technology, we believe, will continue to influence health literacy as it makes information from most sources easier to access and share. At the same time, it challenges individuals to understand and evaluate various sources in order to make effective and appropriate decisions. As Western societies in particular continue to age, policy makers will demand that technology be employed to support patient self-care, especially for seniors and others needing long-term care. The commercial media will continue to be a particularly influential user of technology; health-literate citizens will be increasingly called upon to take a questioning stance when confronted by putative health advice from advertisers (e.g., our diet pill works) or indirectly from video games and television programming (e.g., violent behaviour is fun and risk free). Today's largely technologically focussed adolescents will grow to adulthood expecting more information and support to be available through social media.

Relationship of Health Literacy and Health Policy

Health policy arising from and influencing health literacy, we foresee, will be an ongoing interest of governments and political parties. Populations, in the Western world especially, have strong opinions on the costs and benefits of their health care systems. Politicians will continue to attempt to address and influence public opinion in order to be elected and will adopt policies of 'individual responsibility' or 'social responsibility' according to their party platforms. In addition, the mounting cost of health care, especially given the aging population in most Western countries, will make politicians interested in ways to improve health outcomes while keeping costs down. Economic considerations will give health literacy advocates one of their strongest arguments for government support. This anticipated trend underscores the need for clarity in the definition applied, rigour in measurement tools, and a commitment to the evaluation of health literacy interventions.

Health Inequalities as an Impetus for a More Health-Literate Population

The extent to which governments frame their policies with regard to a concern about growing health inequalities will influence public health practitioners' engagement with health literacy and their work with marginalized populations. Although health literacy has an impact on the capacity for health of individuals from all segments of society, those with less socioeconomic advantage are more likely to have inadequate health literacy and to be harder to reach through conventional services. As the New London Group (1996) pointed out, however, the more skills people possess to understand and communicate in a variety of situations, the more access they will have to the information they need to make appropriate health decisions "creating access to the evolving language of work, power, and community, and fostering the critical engagement necessary for [learners] to design their social futures" (p. 60). Reducing the gap between groups having more and less access to health education and services, and the capacity to act on information received, will continue to be a vitally important function of health literacy in the future.

CONCLUSION

In Chapter 1, we described the emergence of health literacy as "an international phenomenon" (Paasche-Orlow, McCaffery, and Wolf, 2009, p. 293). As authors with various disciplinary and international perspectives remind us, a consideration for context is vital to the future success of health literacy interventions. In their chapters, authors have illustrated the multiple contexts in which health literacy is relevant, including but not limited to different research and practice settings, population groups, stages along the life course, fields of practice, issues of concern, policy positions, and information and service delivery systems. This book demonstrates that the complexity of health literacy necessarily reflects the multiple contexts in which it applies and the perspectives of those who engage with it in their research and practice. Health literacy is a thriving area of interest that, we suggest, will continue to grow in importance as we face health challenges in the future. We hope this book has inspired readers to learn more about health literacy, to contribute as scholars and practitioners to this evolving field, and to become health literacy advocates in whatever contexts they find themselves situated in the future.

Questions for Reflection

1) How does context influence research, policy, and practice in health literacy?
2) What is the value of engaging international perspectives on health literacy?
3) How can health literacy researchers, practitioners, and policy makers promote interdisciplinary collaborations? What might be the challenges and rewards of such collaborations?
4) What are practical ways that you can apply health literacy in schools, clinics, communities, hospitals, or other health contexts?
5) How can health literacy advocates influence policy makers?
6) Which definitions and conceptions of health literacy are most appropriate in your context?

7) What are the key challenges for the future of health literacy? What trends do you foresee?
8) Which chapters are of most interest to your work in health literacy? Why?
9) Do you consider yourself to be a health literacy advocate? Why?
10) Are you health literate?

REFERENCES

Commission on the Social Determinants of Health. (2008). *Closing the gap in a generation: Health equity through action on the social determinants of health (Final Report)*. Geneva, Switzerland: World Health Organization Commission.

European Health Literacy Survey. (2011). *HLS-EU homepage*. Retrieved from http://inthealth.eu/research/health-literacy-hls-eu/.

New London Group. (1996). A pedagogy of multiliteracies: Designing social futures. *Harvard Educational Review, 66*(1), 60-92.

Nielsen-Bohlman, L., Panzer, A. M., and Kindig, D. A. (Eds.). (2004). *Health literacy: A prescription to end confusion*. Washington, DC: Institute of Medicine of the National Academies and The National Academies Press.

Nutbeam, D. (2009). Defining and measuring health literacy: What can we learn from literacy studies? *International Journal of Public Health, 54*, 303-305.

Paasche-Orlow, M. K., McCaffery, K., and Wolf, M. S. (2009). Bridging the international divide for health literacy research. *Patient Education and Counseling, 75*, 293-294.

Rootman, I., and Gordon-El-Bihbety, D. (2008). *A vision for a health literate Canada: Report of the expert panel on health literacy*. Ottawa, Canada: Canadian Public Health Association.

Stableford, S., and Mettger, W. (2007). Plain language: A strategic response to the health literacy challenge. *Journal of Public Health Policy, 28*, 71-93.

Wanless, D. (2002). *Securing our future health: Taking a long-term view*. Retrieved from http://si.easp.es/derechosciudadania/wp-content/uploads/2009/10/4.Informe-Wanless.pdf.

World Health Organization. (1998). *Health promotion glossary*. Geneva, Switzerland: Author.

BIOGRAPHIES OF HEALTH LITERACY BOOK AUTHORS

Deborah L. Begoray is a Professor of Literacy Education at the University of Victoria, British Columbia, Canada. She studies adolescent literacy not only in English language arts classrooms but also in other subject areas such as history, science, and mathematics. Her interest in the literacies needed to succeed in health education classrooms led her to health literacy research. Dr. Begoray has studied the health literacies of Indigenous adolescent girls, among others, and has written on improvements to nursing curricula that might arise from including health literacy practices. Currently, she is working on research examining the relationships between and among health literacy, adolescents, and the media. E-mail: dbegoray@uvic.ca

Diarmuid Coughlan is currently a National Cancer Institute-sponsored Health Economics Visting Fellow at Johns Hopkins School of Public Health, Baltimore, Maryland, USA. His interest in healthcare systems emanated from working as a pharmacist in the UK, Australia, America, and his native Ireland. Moreover, it was his return to academia to study the contribution of community pharmacy to patient education that led him to conduct health literacy themed research. Subsequently, he completed a master's degree in Health Economics at the University of York, England, and his PhD thesis will stress the importance of a health literacy centered healthcare system. E-mail: dcoughla@jhsph.edu

Doris Gillis is an Associate Professor in Human Nutrition at St. Francis Xavier University in Nova Scotia, Canada. Dr. Gillis draws upon her academic and professional background in public health nutrition, health promotion, and adult education in exploring issues related to health literacy, food security, and maternal and child nutrition. She has been involved in a number of community-university research initiatives including leading a participatory research project exploring the links between health and literacy in rural Nova Scotia. She was a member of the Canadian Expert Panel on Health Literacy and continues to be engaged in national efforts to advance health literacy. E-mail: dgillis@stfx.ca

Nicola Gray is is a freelance research consultant based in Manchester, England. A community pharmacist by background, her research and policy interests include health literacy with a focus upon young people's health and medicines information. She is a Trustee of the Association for Young People's Health and a Fellow of the US Society for Adolescent Health and Medicine. Her Harkness Fellowship in 2001-02 in the Division of Adolescent Medicine at the University of Rochester, New York, sparked her interest in health literacy as a framework for exploring the challenges that young people face when searching the Internet for information about health and medicines. E-mail: nicola@webstar.co.uk

Albert Lee is a Professor (Clinical) and Founding Director of the Centre for Health Education and Health Promotion of the School of Public Health and Primary Care of the Chinese University of Hong Kong; he also holds adjunct/visiting professorships in leading academic institutions in the USA, UK, and Australia. He holds a medical degree from the University of London, master and doctorate degrees and professional qualifications in Public Health and Family Medicine at the Fellowship level, as well as a master's degree in Research and Professional Study in Education. He first pioneered the concept of Health Promoting Schools in Hong Kong, and his framework has been widely cited and adopted by many neighbouring countries. Dr. Lee has been invited to serve as a WHO temporary advisor on many occasions on school health, healthy cities, and health promotion. E-mail: alee@cuhk.edu.hk

Diane Levin-Zamir is Director of the National Department of Health Education and Promotion of Clalit, Israel's largest health service organization, and a Lecturer in the Schools of Public Health in Haifa, Tel Aviv, and Hebrew universities. She specializes in action research pertaining to health promotion concerns in community, hospital, and media settings with a particular focus on media health literacy and health literacy measurement. Dr. Levin-Zamir leads the Israel Health Literacy Survey. She has served in numerous leadership roles with the International Union of Health Education and Promotion including on the editorial board of the Global Health Promotion Journal and on global working groups. She is one of the founding members of the Israel Association of Health Promoters and Educators. E-mail: diamos@zahav.net.il

E. Anne Marshall is a Professor of Counselling Psychology and Director of the Centre for Youth and Society, an interdisciplinary research centre at the University of Victoria, British Columbia, Canada. Her research focuses on adolescent and emerging adulthood transitions, mental health, mental health literacy, and cultural identity. Dr. Marshall is co-editor of *Ethical issues in community-based research with children and youth* (2006) and *Knowledge translation in context: Indigenous, policy and community settings* (2011), both published by University of Toronto Press. E-mail: amarshal@uvic.ca

Alexa T. McCray is an Associate Professor of Medicine at Harvard Medical School, Boston, Massachusetts, USA. She is the former Director of the Lister Hill National Center for Biomedical Communications, a research division of the National Library of Medicine at the US National Institutes of Health. Dr. McCray was elected to the Institute of Medicine of the National Academy of Sciences in 2001. She is a fellow of the American Association for the Advancement of Science and a fellow of the American College of Medical Informatics. She is a past member of the boards of both the American Medical Informatics Association and the International Medical Informatics Association. Dr. McCray conducts research in biomedical informatics, including health communication/literacy. E-mail: alexa.mccray@hms. harvard. edu

Don Nutbeam is Vice-Chancellor of the University of Southampton, England, a position he has held since 2009. His career has spanned positions in universities, government, health services, and an independent research institute. From 2003-09, he was in senior academic roles in the University of Sydney, Australia; prior to this, he was Head of Public Health in the UK Department of Health. Professor Nutbeam has substantial international experience in both developing and developed countries, working as an advisor and consultant for the World Health Organisation over a 20-year period and as consultant and team leader in projects for the World Bank. E-mail: vice-chancellor@soton.ac.uk

Joanne Protheroe is a Senior Lecturer in General Practice at Keele University, England, and a practising family doctor in Manchester. Dr. Protheroe's primary research interests include decision aids/decision analysis, facilitating decision making in general practice and disadvantaged groups, and patient participation and health literacy. She has been Deputy Chair of the Health Literacy UK group since 2008 and is now Chair Elect; she currently serves on a Royal College of Physicians working party examining Doctor-Patient Communication. E-mail: j.protheroe@keele.ac.uk

Irving Rootman is an Adjunct Professor at the University of Victoria, British Columbia, Canada. Previously, he was the Executive Director of the Health and Learning Knowledge Centre at the University of Victoria. He served as the Co-Chair of the Canadian Expert Panel on Health Literacy and was a member of the US Institute of Medicine Expert Committee on Health Literacy. Dr. Rootman was a Michael Smith Foundation for Health Research Distinguished Scholar and Professor at the University of Victoria and, prior to that, the founding Director of the Centre for Health Promotion at the University of Toronto. Earlier in his career, he was a researcher, research manager, and program manager for Health and Welfare Canada. Dr. Rootman has published widely on health literacy as well as health promotion. E-mail: irootman@telus.net

Gillian Rowlands is an academic General Practitioner (Family Physician) at the London South Bank University, England. Prof. Rowlands' interest in the field of health literacy was sparked by her recognition of low literacy and numeracy skills as an invisible barrier to patients' understanding about, and ability to improve, their health. The invisibility of low patient-health-literacy skills meant that it is often not recognised, or made allowance for, by practitioners, compounding the difficulties experienced by patients. Her perspective is on how health literacy affects patient-practitioner communication and how the skills of patients and practitioners might be built to empower patients. E-mail: rowlang2@lsbu.ac.uk

Rima Rudd is a faculty member in the Department of Society, Human Development, and Health at the Harvard School of Public Health, Boston, Massachusetts, USA. Dr. Rudd has focused her research and policy work on literacy-related disparities and literacy barriers to health programs, services, and care. She has served on numerous committees including the US Institute of Medicine Committee on Health Literacy, the National Research Council Committee on Measuring Adult Literacy, the Joint Commission Advisory Committee on Health Literacy and Patient Safety, and the Surgeon General's Workshop on Health Literacy. She has written several reports that have helped shape the agenda in health literacy research and practice and is the recipient of numerous awards for her leadership. She serves as a co-principal investigator on several on-going health literacy research projects and collaborates with scholars across the US and in many European countries. E-mail: RRUDD@hsph.harvard.edu

Laura P. Shone is an Associate Professor of Pediatrics, Clinical Nursing, and the Center for Community Health at the University of Rochester Medical Center, New York, USA. Dr Shone's research focuses on the interface between individuals and systems. Examples include health care access, financing, outcomes, and policy for children, adolescents, and young adults. She has conducted extensive research in the areas of child and adolescent health insurance including SCHIP, racial and ethnic disparities. She is currently leading one of the first US-government-funded studies of health literacy to focus on transition-age adolescents and young adults. E-mail: Laura_Shone@URMC.Rochester.edu

Jane Wills is Professor of Health Promotion at London South Bank University, England. She has written extensively on health promotion and been influential in its development as a field of activity over the past 20 years. Her textbooks have been translated into five languages and are on the core curricula of nursing and health studies in many countries. She has been co-editor of *Critical Public Health* and regularly lectures at universities in Europe, Africa, and Australia. She is part of a research Institute for Primary Care and Public Health where her work focuses on local and national work to discover what works and for whom in building health and wellbeing. E-mail: willsj@lsbu.ac.uk

Michael S. Wolf is an Associate Professor of Medicine, Associate Division Chief of Research, and Director of the Health Literacy and Learning Program in the Feinberg School of Medicine at Northwestern University, Evanston, Illinois, USA. Dr. Wolf is a cognitive/behavioral scientist and health services researcher who publishes widely on adult literacy and learning, human factors, and the management of chronic disease. He is a Fulbright Distinguished Faculty Scholar (UK) and currently serves on advisory committees for the US Food and Drug Administration, US Pharmacopeia, the American Dental Association, and the Agency for Healthcare Research and Quality. E-mail: mswolf@northwestern.edu

INDEX

G

F

H

I

S

T